D1054463

The

Breast Cancer

Survival Manual

*why every week instead of
every 3 weeks?
effect on white cell count*

280-8884

JOHN LINK, M.D.

The
BREAST
CANCER

· SURVIVAL MANUAL ·

A Step-by-Step Guide
for the Woman with Newly
Diagnosed Breast Cancer

SECOND EDITION

AN OWL BOOK

HENRY HOLT AND COMPANY · NEW YORK

Henry Holt and Company, LLC
Publishers since 1866
115 West 18th Street
New York, New York 10011

Henry Holt® is a registered trademark of Henry Holt and Company, LLC.
Copyright © 1998, 2000 by John Link, M.D.
All rights reserved.
Published in Canada by Fitzhenry & Whiteside Ltd.,
195 Allstate Parkway, Markham, Ontario L3R 4T8.

Library of Congress Cataloging-in-Publication Data

Link, John, M.D.
The breast cancer survival manual : a step-by-step guide for the
woman with newly diagnosed breast cancer / John Link—2nd ed.
p.   cm.
"An owl book."
Includes bibliographical references and index.
ISBN 0-8050-6400-1 (pbk.)
1. Breast—Cancer—Popular works.   I. Title.
RC280.B8 L53   2000   99-047515
616.99′449—dc21

Henry Holt books are available for special promotions and
premiums. For details contact: Director, Special Markets.

Second Edition 2000

Printed in the United States of America

1 3 5 7 9 10 8 6 4 2

To my wife, Victoria,
and my four daughters,
Erin, Ashley,
Amanda, and Brittany,
and to the cure of
breast cancer

Nothing in life is to be feared.
It is only to be understood.
—Marie Curie

Contents

Acknowledgments

This manual was conceived as a teaching guide for the women with newly diagnosed breast cancer who come to our breast center. I want to thank Diane Vuoso Munz for the countless hours she spent making the dream a reality. Thank you to Melissa Miller Jeffries for being my right hand, tirelessly managing one project after another.

The medical care of women with breast cancer is a team effort, and I have had the privilege of being on several outstanding teams at the Memorial Breast Centers in Southern California. The nurses at Long Beach—Lisa Kemp, Pattie Proffitt, Carolyn Amberry, Patti Brown, Susan Tanaka, and Patty Donnelly—have helped develop, and put into practice on a daily basis, the best standards of exceptional care. I would particularly like to acknowledge Julio Ibarra and Lowell Rogers, superb breast pathologists; Arthur Diamond, Susan Roux, Debra Butler, and Brooke Caldwell, dedicated breast radiologists; Tomi Evans, Cary Kaufman, Pamela Craig, and Jim Wells, wonderful surgeons; and Cynthia Forsthoff, my associate and outstanding medical oncologist. The team also includes psychotherapist Lisa Donley, nutrition specialist Kami Lakis, and Nancy Barnett, an expert in oriental medicine. Nancy's wisdom and knowledge picked up where my medical school training left off.

I thank Claudia Lee and Cathy Coleman for their vision and support throughout the years. A special thanks to Andrea Martin, president of the Breast Cancer Fund. I also must recognize and thank Kim Granger and the Patricia A. Brown Trust for their support of the "Breast Friends" program, for which this manual was initially conceived.

Certainly, my most influential and greatest teacher has been László Tabár, and I am forever appreciative. I have great admiration for Bernard Fisher, M.D., who pioneered breast cancer clinical research in this country. As a medical student, I was greatly influenced by Loren Stephens, who helped me appreciate the complexity of the human being. Special thanks to Randi and Greg Gunther: to Randi for her friendship, knowledge, and advice over the years, and to Greg for his assistance with the illustrations in the manual.

I have the good fortune and privilege to go to work each day and work with people I enjoy and respect. I would particularly like to recognize David Delgado, CEO of Breastlink Medical Group, for his talent, loyalty, and service.

There are two women who have influenced the course of breast cancer care in this country and have helped bring women into the decision-making process. Many thanks to Rose Kushner and Wendy Schain. I would also like to thank my agent, Sheree Bykofsky, and Amelia Sheldon of Henry Holt for their support.

Last, but most important, I want to thank the women I have had the privilege to care for.

The
Breast Cancer
Survival Manual

Introduction
About This Manual

This book is a crisis manual. It is an attempt to put into writing what we do on a daily basis, which is to help women with newly diagnosed breast cancer understand their situation and develop a plan to optimize a cure. With this life-threatening and certainly life-changing diagnosis, we ask women to become immediately educated and make critical decisions. We, the medical profession, demand this at a time of immense crisis in a woman's life—a time of fear, confusion, and panic. It's not fair. During this time of crisis, women need a direct, informative, honest approach to the choices they are being asked to make about the management of their newly diagnosed cancer.

In my daily practice, I encounter women from all walks of life who are given the diagnosis of breast cancer. Regardless of their background, they experience similar emotions: shock, denial, panic, and a sense of urgency. Most of these women are in no position to rush into treatment. They lack the information and education that are crucial for making sound decisions about their medical care.

This sense of urgency dates back to the old way of treating breast cancer, prior to 1970, when the "one stage" mastectomy, or removal of the entire breast, was "the" treatment. Breast cancer treatment today involves surgery, radiation, chemotherapy, and hormones; the sequencing of these treatments may vary depending on a woman's situation. In a majority of cases, we can have a preoperative diagnosis based on a needle biopsy. Needle biopsies can be performed on small, nonpalpable (cannot be felt) lesions using image-guided assistance with either an ultrasound machine or a mammogram. Palpable lesions can also be biopsied with a needle, so that the woman usually knows her diagnosis before undergoing any surgery.

The first information I give a patient is that there *is time*—usually several weeks to a month—to confirm the diagnosis, seek expert opinions, and develop a survival plan. By taking this extra time to come up with a treatment plan, a woman will be incurring minimal risk and may very well have an enhanced chance of cure.

Taking a little time is very helpful because now the "right approach" can be planned without "burning any bridges." In other words, some treatment decisions made now cannot be undone at a later time. Some women need very limited surgery without the removal of the lymph nodes in the armpit (axilla). Other women may need treatment with chemotherapy prior to any operation. Since the treatment of breast cancer may involve multiple specialists such as a breast surgeon, plastic surgeon, radiation oncologist, medical oncologist, pathologist, and radiologist, it is also important to use a coordinated approach with a team leader. I will address the development of a plan and picking the team in chapter 7.

The old method of treating women with breast cancer was what I call the sequential method, in which a woman would see a succession of specialists, usually beginning with the surgeon. Each physician would then do what his or her training dictated. For instance, a surgeon operates, a radiation oncologist irradiates, and a chemotherapist gives chemotherapy. The newer approach integrates treatment and has the different doctors working together in concert. Clearly, this is what the woman wants: her various treating physicians communicating with each other and working as a team toward a uniform treatment plan.

Unfortunately, medicine has become so specialized that physicians are now basically trained to perform only specific treatments. To paraphrase Abraham Maslow, renowned psychologist, if all you have is a hammer, then all you do is drive nails. So it is very important that there is someone on the team who understands and has an overview of the total treatment of breast cancer and who can coordinate the various tests and treatments. This team leader could be any one of your treating doctors, but there must be a mutual understanding that this physician is assuming the role.

With recent changes in health care delivery, many women may have difficulty finding someone who can coordinate their care. In managed care situations, choices may differ from the private-practice model. If you are in a health maintenance organization (HMO), you can receive "state of the art" therapy, but it is critical that you become well educated and play a leading role in directing your care. You may need to go outside your HMO for a second opinion. Some managed care organizations will pay for this, although it may take some assertiveness on your part. In chapter 1, we will cover how and when to get an appropriate second opinion. This may add an extra week before actual treatment can begin, *but it will be time well spent.*

I would like also to strongly emphasize that breast cancer is a heterogeneous disease. Breast cancer has a tremendous variability in the way it presents itself, the way it looks under the microscope, the way it behaves biologically, and the way it interacts within each individual woman. These factors are extremely important in planning therapy.

Both the lay public and the medical profession tend to simplify breast cancer and make it homogeneous so that the treatment can be standardized. Although we know that breast cancer has a number of commonalities, that does not justify using the same treatment for every woman. We've come a long way since the 1950s, when the only treatment was a radical mastectomy. We now have a much better understanding of local control and the factors that affect cancer's spread into the lymph and blood systems. Consider your individual uniqueness regarding this disease and its treatment, and understand that it is important not to see yourself or let your treatment team see you as a statistic.

If you believe you are becoming a statistic in their eyes and feel you are being categorized into stages and outcome probabilities based on information from women who have preceded you with this disease, you may not get the best treatment for you. Such an experience can be dehumanizing, if it happens, and it can lead to a negative outcome. Our rapidly evolving knowledge base and technological development allow for a much more individualized approach, which can be more effective for you and your particular situation. You should be sure to feel that your treatment takes full advantage of this.

Clearly, we should attempt to "fingerprint" each woman's cancer in order to make the best treatment choices. This fingerprinting allows us to look at a number of characteristics including size of tumor, cell of origin, growth behavior, hormone influence, ability to invade lymph and blood vessels, and genetic changes. Don't worry, this is not as complex as it may sound to you now. Most of this information is available from your mammograms and the biopsy, and you will have a better understanding of how to use the information after reading this manual.

To treat breast cancer without considering the woman herself is a tremendous mistake. A woman's age, her hormone status, her general health, her emotional support network, her sexuality, her immune system, and her psychological and spiritual being—all are important in planning her treatment and maintaining her health. Because traditional medicine has often neglected to treat the whole person, many women today are seeking out "complementary therapy." Sadly, I see a few women who are so distrustful of traditional medical treatment that they have used only alternative therapies. These women come back to conventional medicine months to years later with advanced breast cancer and in a state of crisis. An ideal treatment plan should consider the benefits of nutrition, vitamins, certain herbs, psychotherapy, physical therapy, as well as the best that medicine has to offer.

I start this manual with a chapter on second opinions. It may seem strange to you, discussing a second opinion at the very same time you are coping with your first opinion. Although I stated earlier that there is time to educate yourself regarding your cancer, second opinions can take a few weeks to obtain and may even involve a trip to a major cancer facility. Because of the confusion and element of denial you will be facing as a newly diagnosed cancer patient, it is often recommended that you seek second opinions so you are confident with your diagnosis and treatment plan before initiating your treatment. It is also important to put this chapter up front because there has been much discussion in the lay literature about getting second opinions. Many women and their families feel anxious or guilty about asking the diagnosing physician to help gather materials and records to give to another physician or institution for a second opinion. You need not worry about this.

After considering the issue of a second opinion, I provide basic information, in chapters 2, 3, 4, and 5, on the nature and biology of breast cancer and how they affect your overall treatment plan. In chapter 4, I discuss in some depth how to analyze your pathology report and the importance of this information in planning your treatment. Accurate interpretation of what the cancer looks like under the microscope is absolutely critical. This important information needs to be confirmed by the physician rendering a second opinion. Chapter 5 deals with the various types of breast cancer, and chapter 6 is devoted to ductal cancer in situ (DCIS), an early cancer that accounts for up to 20 percent of newly diagnosed breast cancer.

Chapter 7 deals with the selection of an appropriate treatment team to care for you and provides helpful tips on how you can choose someone who will take charge and coordinate the individual team members. In the following chapters, I offer more details on the issues surrounding actual treatment methods such as radiation, chemotherapy, and hormone therapies such as tamoxifen. At this point I discuss the purpose of clinical research trials and how they might affect you and your treatment. I then move on to the important issue of complementary care, considering the place of diet and herbs, and the connection between your emotional state and your cancer prognosis.

Many women who have daughters are concerned about genetic risk and testing. So in chapter 15, I discuss the genetics of breast cancer, testing, and the future risk of developing breast cancer. Once you have gone through this whole ordeal, you may have a certain amount of anxiety about moving on with your life. New medical concerns may arise after treatment, and even in their absence, the fear of recurrence is quite common. These issues are addressed in chapters 16 and 17.

Chapter 18 explains how to get the best medical care available by discussing the dos and don'ts of dealing with personnel in different medical systems.

Chapter 19 shows you how to keep a diary and a log as well as an overall treatment calendar, and why it is a good idea to develop the habit of organizing your medical records. Taking charge of your own medical records can make your doctor visits more productive and actually ensure that you get optimal care.

It is my hope that this manual will be helpful to you during a difficult period. The last ten years of my cancer medical practice have been devoted to women with breast cancer, and I have seen the positive effects that patient participation in forming a treatment plan has had. Since more and more physicians today are asking for their patients' help with the important decisions regarding treatment, you need to have the proper preparation to become an informed participant in the decision-making process.

Keep in mind that most women are fearful that their recommended therapy is inadequate. This is particularly true of women coming from managed care organizations. Of equal concern, however, is overtreatment. Many women are being overtreated without understanding the true risks, benefits, and appropriateness of the therapy they receive. I hope to help alleviate those fears by clearly describing all the options open to you.

The main objective of this book is to give you some control over what may seem like chaos. Information and knowledge are critical and constantly changing. You will have access to the latest information on the treatment of breast cancer through the Internet; see the "Resources" section at the back of the book for a number of important Web sites. Although I have been updating the material in this book on a continuing basis, publication will stop the process. To continue to provide you with current information, I will update this manual through the Internet (at http://www.breastlinkcare.com).

I recommend that you use this book as a manual or workbook. Underline and make notes in the margins. Consider, as I suggest in chapter 19, making a companion three-ring binder of your own personal information, including reports, logs, and calendars.

But whether you skim it once or it never leaves your side throughout your treatment, I hope when you do put this book down it will have informed and empowered you, helping you to receive the best cancer treatment and care that is *right for you* at this time in history.

1
......

Second Opinions

Why is it important to get a second opinion when you have been diagnosed with breast cancer? There are several reasons.

Even when you trust your physicians completely, the gravity of a cancer diagnosis demands that you feel fully confident with the diagnosis and your treatment plan before proceeding any further. A second opinion that concurs with the first can give you that confidence.

Although confirmation is comforting, a second opinion can also add to or conflict with information you may have already received. But even conflicting data can set up a productive dialogue that leads to a more appropriate treatment plan and a better understanding of your situation.

Also, because of managed care, some women are given little choice in selecting physicians or treatment options, and they want to make sure their medical system will do the right thing. A second consultation can provide the diagnostic support to help them obtain the appropriate care.

Our center renders several hundred second opinions a year to women with newly diagnosed breast cancer who have come to us from other facilities. We also diagnose several hundred women with breast cancer every year in our own breast center. Even though we are regarded as experts in the field, we understand a woman's need to hear confirmation from another source. In any way we can, we encourage and will facilitate a second opinion for any of our patients. I feel it is extremely important that each patient be comfortable with and have confidence in her treatment team. I welcome outside opinions before embarking on a course of therapy. Occasionally, new information is brought forth from another source, or a different approach is presented that is better suited to the patient.

You should not be afraid or hesitant about requesting a second opinion; nor should a doctor be concerned about your receiving one. On the contrary, this process should be encouraged, and any center or physician that discourages it should be willing to discuss with you their reasons for not supporting you on this very important issue.

A good second opinion takes time and costs money—about $500. It includes an independent review of the cancerous tissue by a pathologist, a review of X rays and imaging studies by a breast radiologist, and presentation to a treatment team for a proposed plan. This process requires the integration of a team of experienced experts. The second opinion is usually enlightening, solidifying information you have already obtained from your diagnosing doctor and from your own independent research. Occasionally, the second opinion differs drastically from the first, placing you in a dilemma. If the institution rendering the differing opinion is experienced and reputable, the medical team will explain the basis of this opinion to you and your other physicians.

Sometimes, a third opinion is necessary and should be rendered by a center specializing in breast cancer treatment. Our center has seen women who are seeking a fourth or even fifth opinion. Additional opinions beyond the third will usually differ little and will only delay your decision regarding a treatment plan.

The second opinion process should be started as soon as you have made the decision to seek it. Often, your diagnosing facility or doctor can be helpful in recommending a regional facility that specializes in breast cancer treatment. This may be a university, a large urban hospital, or a private facility. The process of securing another doctor's or team's opinion involves several steps and may take a week or more to complete. Often a second opinion requires the physician to review your pathological material and imaging studies, usually before you are seen.

The purpose of the second opinion is to get a comprehensive, independent review of your cancer. Reports and records are not enough. As noted earlier, the cancerous tissue must be examined (under the microscope), and the X rays and other images reviewed. You should be interviewed and given a complete history and physical examination. Based on all of the information, the experts should present you with treatment options and explain the inherent risks and benefits of those options.

The price you pay for this time and expertise will be money well spent. Keep in mind that most insurance companies require you to take your automobile to several auto body repair shops for estimates before they are willing to pay to have the work done. Your life is certainly worth more than your automobile, and you deserve the highest standard of care.

You should feel confident your diagnosis is correct, and comfortable with the suggested treatment. Remember, mistakes can happen, and there can be areas of disagreement and differences in treatment style. Some facilities, for example, will treat 80 percent of the women they see with mastectomies for local control. In another facility, it may be 20 percent, with the same cure rate at both locations. Why the difference? For the most part, physicians, like people everywhere, have different ways of approaching a problem and believe that what they are doing is best and have their reasons for their treatment choices. You must consider the opinions presented to you and choose the treatment plan that you feel is right for you.

There is a good chance that your second opinion will simply confirm the diagnosis and treatment suggested by your own doctor. From your first and second opinions and the reading and research you have done, you now are ready to settle on a treatment team and develop a comprehensive treatment plan. This may be hard for you to believe, but you can reach this point in a two- to three-week period. While you may think you will never be able to decide on your own treatment, you may be pleasantly surprised. In the upcoming weeks, you will find that your confidence and desire to participate in your own care will increase with the amount of information and guidance you have. It is not a path you would have chosen but one you must take, and the better prepared you are, the safer the trip.

If you decide to seek a second opinion, which I highly recommend, here are some suggestions to guide you through the process:

- Inform your primary physician and/or your diagnosing physician that you are considering another opinion. Ask for his/her help in suggesting a facility and getting your records and material ready to bring to the second facility. Some women seek a second opinion prior to really receiving a full first opinion, which I discourage you from doing. It is important to know what your "home physician team" recommends before getting the second or outside opinion. If your diagnosing doctor and his/her colleagues are reluctant to share their conclusions with you, ask them why they feel this way and make certain the reasons are in *your* best interest.
- Select a doctor, breast cancer center, or hospital to approach. There is a large network of breast cancer survivors who are glad to offer information and discuss their personal experiences with different medical facilities. Organizations such as the local American Cancer Society, National Cancer Institute, and the Y-Me Support Group can also help provide information. In addition, the Internet is becoming an increasingly valuable resource for information. And for misinformation as well, unless it's an established organization's site. For additional names and phone numbers, turn to the "Resources" section of this book.
- Contact the facility you have selected for the second opinion. Ask questions when making your appointment over the phone. Find

out the name of the person with whom you are speaking and what role that individual plays in the process. You will usually talk to a nurse or trained medical assistant. He or she should explain the process of getting a second opinion at his/her facility, what information is needed, and how you can facilitate the evaluation. Oftentimes, rather than having the second facility request your records from your doctor and hospital, it is preferable to pick up your slides and X rays yourself and hand-deliver them to the facility that is rendering the second opinion. This gives you an opportunity to see the facility and helps ensure that your records do not get misplaced. If there is a distance factor and the material needs to be sent, you may want to pick up your slides and X rays and send them via an overnight courier that has tracking capabilities to guarantee that they get there in a timely manner. You have some time, but you don't want to waste time.

- Go into this facility for an opinion *only*. Do not approach it as a treatment facility. After you have processed all the information, you may decide to seek treatment at the facility where you received your second opinion, but that is not your primary goal at this point. You want honest, accurate information you can use. If this treatment facility has a dual agenda, such as entering you in an experimental protocol for which it is being funded, try to keep that issue separate from the matter of the second opinion. Let the staff know you are initially visiting just for a second opinion.

- Make sure you are receiving accurate information regarding your diagnosis and the best advice on treatment planning. I am often asked by patients or their spouses, "Doctor, if this were your wife, what would you recommend?" The very nature of the question implies a double standard in the medical profession. The assumption is that the physician would treat a patient one way but might do something different for a family member. Unfortunately, to varying degrees, this double standard can exist, and with "managed care" becoming more prevalent, there is even more reason for you to be vigilant about your medical care. In fact, in a recent study conducted by epidemiologists at the University of California, Irvine, breast cancer treatment differences and outcomes were observed in Orange County, California, between 1984 and 1990. Women treated at small nonteaching hospitals and HMOs had a much higher mastectomy rate and significantly decreased survival rate.* This type of data underscores how important it is for you to gather as much information as possible and be your own advocate.

· Be prepared for the second opinion outcome. While you are waiting for your appointment, you have time to educate yourself. This manual will help, as will other resources listed in the back. You will need to know how to read the pathology report and identify the important information (chapter 4). You should have a list of questions ready for the doctor, and I suggest that you ask if you may audiotape the session. At our center, we actually do this for all of the women who seek second opinions from us. It has been our experience that women only retain part of what is said at the appointment, due to both the amount of information given and the mental anguish they may be suffering as a result of their recent cancer diagnosis. Sometimes, women have recently gone off replacement hormones, and their cognitive function is temporarily impaired as well. In addition to audiotaping, you might consider bringing a loved one along to the session, as some women find that having extra support during the appointment is reassuring.

CHECKPOINTS

1. Would I feel more comfortable getting another opinion before beginning the suggested treatment?
2. Should I go out of town or stay local for a second opinion? Out of town opinions are often less threatening to your home team.

---

*Anna Lee-Feldstein et al., "Treatment Differences and Other Prognostic Factors Related to Breast Cancer Survival," JAMA 271, no. 15 (1994): 1163–68.

3. If I am in an HMO, will the second opinion be paid for by the HMO, or will I need to pay for this out of pocket? Many managed care systems have prearranged contracts for second opinions with a regional center or university. This might be what you are looking for; on the other hand, a referral to another physician within the HMO might not be adequate.

2

Local Control
Surgery and Radiation

If you are like most women in the crisis of newly diagnosed breast cancer, the most immediate and pressing issue is the removal of the cancer from your breast. This chapter deals with these issues of local control. You may feel a tremendous urgency to get the cancer out *now*, but as I have already stated, it is important to take time to develop a pretreatment plan. I use the term *pretreatment* plan because planning should ideally occur before any surgical procedure is done. Breast cancer doctors have spent the last thirty years proving that there are treatment choices regarding local control, and your physicians may very well ask you to help in deciding what is the best treatment for you. In order for you to make informed choices, you need to review some basic biology about breast cancer.

Breast cancer begins with a mutation of a single glandular cell in the breast. The cause or causes for this change in the cell are unknown. Several mutations may occur before the cell is on an irreversible path of uncontrolled replication and growth—the process we call cancer.

Once this event has occurred, cancer cells multiply within the breast. The rate of division and rapidity of growth vary with each cancer. The fastest-growing cancer cells may divide every thirty days, and the slower cancers may take two hundred days or more to replicate.

Cancers stay localized in the breast until they reach a critical size, which we think is, at the very least, 1 cm³ (one cubic centimeter), or one billion cancer cells. Some cancers never develop the ability to spread via the blood or lymph system, no matter how big they get. Figure 2.1 reveals a schematic timeline of cancer cells growing at a rate of division every thirty days.

You will notice that a long period of time elapses before the cancer reaches the critical size that is associated with potential spread into the vascular system. Therefore, when discussing breast cancer treatment, we must address both local control, which is confined to the breast, and the possibility of the cancer's spread into the blood system, which we refer to as systemic control.

The female breast has between ten and twenty separate duct systems, and each duct system converges at the nipple. These duct systems are supported by connective tissue and fat. Each duct system branches into thousands of terminal buds called terminal ductal lobular units (Figure 2.2).

As can be seen from the illustration, there are two basic types of cells in the terminal ductal lobular unit, both of which can potentially

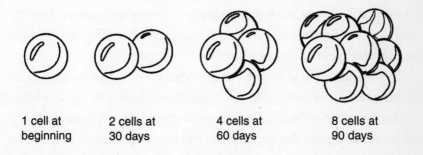

| 1 cell at beginning | 2 cells at 30 days | 4 cells at 60 days | 8 cells at 90 days |

FIGURE 2.1

How cancer cells grow

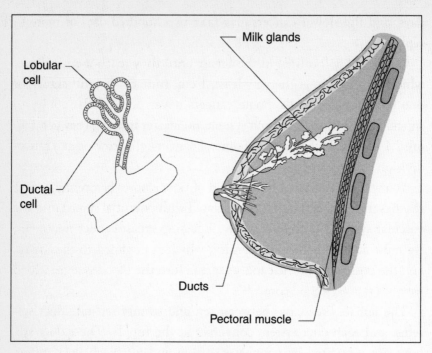

FIGURE 2.2

Breast ducts and lobular cells

mutate and lead to breast cancer: the lobular cell, which is at the terminal bud; and the ductal cell, which lines the entry to the terminal ductal lobular unit. Cancer originating from the lobular cell accounts for about 15 percent of all breast cancers. Cancer originating from the ductal cell accounts for the other 85 percent. The behavior of these two cellular types of cancer is somewhat different.

The ductal type of breast cancer begins when the involved cell makes its cancerous or malignant change, and begins to divide abnormally. The next generation of cells can grow into the duct itself and continue to divide, not penetrating the basement membrane, which acts as a boundary between the ducts and the underlying supportive tissue (see Figure 2.3). Cancers that do not go beyond the basement membrane are called in situ or ductal cancer in situ (DCIS).

When a cancer is in situ, it has not penetrated into the surrounding tissue, blood, or lymph vessels. Cells that grow in the duct tube, termed intraductal cells, are trapped and can continue along the duct system, which eventually leads to the nipple and outside the body. Perhaps 15 to 20 percent of breast cancers are detected in this stage and can remain in this preinvasive phase for some time. These are for the most part "silent" cancers without symptoms, except for a rare bloody nipple discharge or the appearance of calcifications on a mammogram. These small "flecks" of calcium that show up on the mammogram are petrified clumps of dead intraductal cancer cells.

Although in situ breast cancer is not life threatening at this stage, these cells have the ability to continue to divide and spread up and down this ductal "freeway system" and possibly eventually invade the breast tissue beyond the basement membrane.

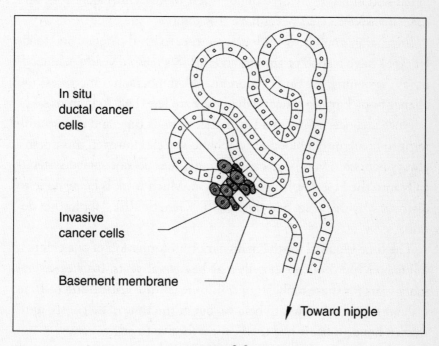

FIGURE 2.3

In situ and invasive ductal cancer

DCIS is a disease that we have recently become aware of because prior to mammographic screening, it was undetectable. Treatment for DCIS is complex and changing. For those of you with DCIS, chapter 5 will address the specific management of this preinvasive cancer.

A ductal cancer cell becomes invasive when it penetrates the basement membrane, the thin mortar that separates the duct from the underlying tissue on the inside of the body. At first, this cancer is microinvasive, which means it can only be seen under the microscope; but with time, it becomes a larger, invasive tumor. As it gains in size and further mutates or changes, it may penetrate not only the basement membrane but also the wall of a lymphatic or blood vessel and escape into the blood system or lymphatic drainage system, markedly increasing the likelihood of metastatic disease, which is a life-threatening event. Breast cancers do not usually spread into the blood system if the invasive tumor is less than 1 cm (Figure 2.4), and some invasive cancers never have this ability.

In general, small invasive breast cancers (both the ductal and lobular type) have a good prognosis, and, for this reason, yearly mammography screening is very important. Mammography increases the chance of picking up cancers when they are less than 1 cm in size.

Once a cancer grows to a larger size, there is time and opportunity for it to break into a blood or lymphatic vessel. However, this doesn't always happen. Even large cancers sometimes do not spread systemically into the blood or lymphatic system. Much work is being done to discover why this is so. See chapter 15, "Genetic Risk," for further details.

The time required for the malignant transformation of one cell to a millimeter (mm) of cancer cells may be several years. It takes several more years for these replicating cells to reach the critical size of 1 cm (10 mm). It may be hard to believe, but at the time of diagnosis, most women have probably had their cancer for five to eight years.

Ductal breast cancers fall into three categories that have "local" treatment implications:

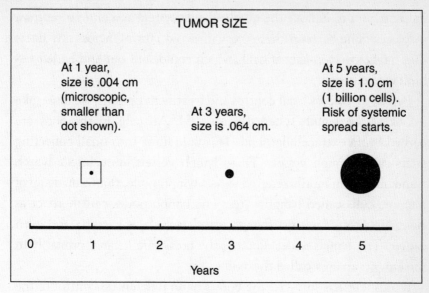

FIGURE 2.4

Tumor growth to one centimeter

1. Ductal cancer in situ, or DCIS (no invasion seen through base-ment membranes)
2. Invasive ductal cancer
3. Invasive ductal cancer with significant in situ component (known as extensive intraductal component, or EIC)

The important distinction regarding ductal cancers occurs when there is ductal cancer in situ (DCIS) present, either alone or associated with invasive cancer. Cancer can spread throughout the ductal system in a diffuse or scattered manner. This diffuse spread of the cancer makes local control more difficult with limited surgery.

In cases such as this, the surgeon must completely remove the area of involved breast tissue and give special attention to the anatomical positioning of the ducts and their relationship to the nipple. To have the best chance of surgically clearing the cancer completely, the surgeon must attempt to remove the involved duct system as a unit rather than in pieces. The surgeon therefore will avoid cutting across any ducts that might contain cancer cells, which could spill out and be left behind in the body.

Before we discuss local control and treatment options, we must take a look at the lymph system (Figure 2.5). All cells in the body are bathed by an extracellular fluid. This fluid flows into small collecting ducts called lymph vessels. These lymph vessels drain into a lymph gland, more commonly referred to as a lymph node, that is made up of immune cells called lymphocytes. The lymph nodes can then act as guards to protect against foreign invaders such as bacteria and even cancer. The lymph nodes draining the breast are located primarily in the armpit, an area called the axilla.

If a cancer has survived the body's natural defenses, control of the cancer must be achieved at the breast site where it originates. This is called local control. Local control is the treatment of the cancer in the breast and the regional lymph system so that it never returns. It is important to understand that even when local control is achieved, cells may have already escaped into the blood system. We refer to this as systemic spread or metastasis. Systemic spread and its control are discussed in detail in chapter 3.

In the first half of this century, the only treatment for the local control of breast cancer was mastectomy, the removal of all possible breast glandular tissue, skin, nipple, and in some instances, the adjacent muscles. The mastectomy originated in the premammography era, when most breast cancers were found as a palpable mass and were much larger and more advanced than the average breast cancer found today.

Clinical trials began forty years ago using less extensive surgery. This surgery is a wide local excision (WLE), also known as a lumpectomy. (Throughout the manual, I will be using the term *wide local excision* exclusively. Wide local excision and lumpectomy are often used interchangeably. A lumpectomy is basically a WLE. A WLE includes removal of breast tissue regardless of whether a lump has been present.

Often there is only a mammographic abnormality with no palpable lump. In this way, the term lumpectomy, although commonly used, can be misleading.) The surgery involves removing the lump or mass along with an area of normal surrounding tissue, achieving what we call a clear margin in which no cancer cells are seen. In spite of achieving clear surgical margins with WLE, the researchers found that the rate of local relapse, in which the cancer returned to the breast, was unacceptable. As a result, trials began adding radiation in conjunction

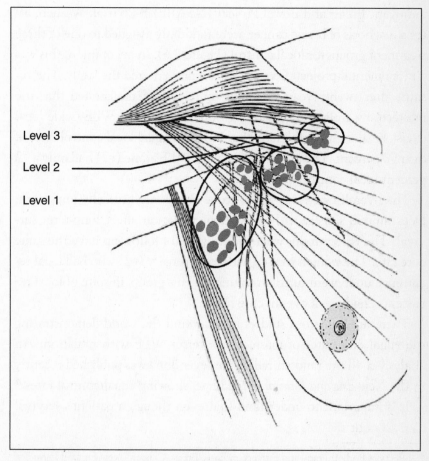

FIGURE 2.5

Distribution of axillary lymph nodes

with this breast conservation surgery. The success of this treatment equaled that seen in women treated with mastectomy alone.

To demonstrate to physicians, and women, that the cure rate with breast conservation surgery in conjunction with radiation therapy was equal to the mastectomy cure rate, the researchers conducted a number of randomized clinical trials. Women bravely agreed to be randomly assigned to either mastectomy or breast conservation treatment and were then followed carefully for local control.

In the 1970s, a large group of cancer physicians conducted one such trial in the United States. The trial was called the National Surgical Adjuvant Breast and Bowel Project (NSABP) B-06 trial. Women, after a diagnosis of breast cancer, were randomly assigned to one of three treatment groups for local control (Figure 2.6). In my opinion, this was a monumental project. Over 2,000 women entered the study. The results, after twenty years of follow-up, clearly demonstrated that the mastectomy group (#1) and the group that received WLE (wide local excision) along with the radiation (#3) had equal local control rates of over 90 percent. The group treated with WLE alone (#2) had only a 72 percent local control rate.

The overall *cure* rates of the three groups are critically important. Does limited surgery with or without radiation affect long-term survival? The three groups with twenty years of follow-up have the same cure rate. The women treated with local surgery (#2) who had local recurrence underwent further treatment. This group, in spite of local recurrence, had equal overall cure rates.

There are numerous studies from around the world demonstrating the equal cure rates of mastectomy versus WLE with radiation. An analysis of all the randomized studies ever done was published recently in the *New England Journal of Medicine*, showing equal control rates.*

It is important to understand that even though a patient's survival

---

* "Effects of Radiotherapy and Surgery in Early Breast Cancer," *New England Journal of Medicine* 333, no. 22 (1995): 1444–55.

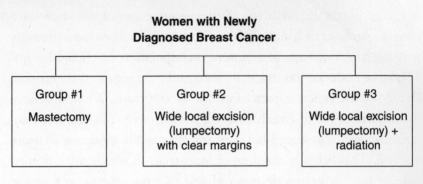

FIGURE 2.6

Three treatment groups in the NSABP B-06 trial

often depends upon whether or not cells have escaped into the vascular system, it is critical for any treatment plan to adequately achieve local control. If this is not done, a woman will be faced with recurrence of cancer in the breast at a later date. While these so-called local recurrences may not ultimately affect cure or survival, they are extremely devastating to the patient psychologically, and they often require more aggressive or extensive surgery and all of the risk involved with it. This has led to the prevailing recommendation that women undergoing wide local excision should follow it up with radiation therapy to help prevent recurrence.

There are situations when mastectomy is performed for local control and, because of the extent of the cancer, radiation treatment is recommended to the mastectomy site. This is often the case when there is extensive involvement of the lymph system. As I will address later in this chapter, if this situation is recognized early, prior to definitive surgery, many treatment centers will recommend chemotherapy to be given first. This presurgical chemotherapy often shrinks the cancer and allows for surgical removal with less than mastectomy. Along with the debate about mastectomy versus wide local excision, another controversial treatment issue is the removal of axillary lymph nodes. The current thinking is that the spread of cancer to the lymph nodes is a very important predictor of the systemic spread of cancer in a patient. Analysis of lymph node involvement has been used to justify systemic therapy, such as hormone manipulation or chemotherapy. The more nodes containing malignant cells, the greater the statistical chance of the cancer's spread into the bloodstream. We now believe that the removal of lymph nodes has value in predicting the likelihood of systemic spread but does not necessarily influence ultimate survival. This belief is based on clinical trials in which some women did not have lymph node removal and had no increase in systemic spread.

To test the effectiveness of lymph node removal, several large clinical trials were performed comparing women who had their lymph nodes removed with women who did not. Both groups underwent lumpectomy and radiation. The two groups had equal overall cure rates, suggesting that metastatic disease caused by the spread of the cancer into the bloodstream occurred primarily in the breast at the site of the original cancer and not through the lymph system.

As more surgeons take note of these results, we are seeing fewer lymph node removals in women with small invasive cancer in which the risk of systemic spread is minimal. Doctors are performing fewer lymph node surgeries on women over the age of seventy with cancer who would not be candidates for chemotherapy under any circumstance. (This is because the more toxic types of chemotherapy are tolerated poorly by elderly women, and the survival benefit is negated by the decreased quality of life. The drug tamoxifen, on the other hand, has minimal toxicity and is almost always the systemic treatment of choice for elderly women.) Also, women who can avoid extensive lymph node removal surgery have less chance of having rare but serious side effects such as nerve damage and lymphatic obstruction (lymphedema of the arm).

There is another comforting piece of data for women who do not have axillary lymph nodes removed. For the rare woman who does later develop a cancerous lymph node, it can be removed without jeopardizing her survival.

Each woman must consider the risks and benefits in choosing breast conservation versus mastectomy. There are rare cases in which a breast conservation including radiation is completely inadvisable. For example, women with collagen vascular diseases—such as systemic lupus, scleroderma, rheumatoid arthritis, or "mixed collagen vascular" disease—should not be treated with radiation. Fortunately, these diseases are quite rare, and women who have them are almost always aware of the diagnosis. The common problem with these diseases is they all involve a vasculitis, which is a disease of small blood vessels that if exposed to radiation can create a severe tissue reaction leading to ulceration and scarring.

Nonrheumatoid types of arthritis such as degenerative arthritis or osteoarthritis are *not* contraindications to radiation. The difference between a collagen vascular disease and the much more common osteoarthritis is usually quite obvious to the treating doctors, and specialized blood tests are extremely helpful in unclear cases. If you have any questions about this, ask your radiation oncologist and physician for advice.

Today, the cosmetic result is good to excellent in 80 to 90 percent of women who receive radiation. Ten percent of women undergoing radiation will have significant skin changes or shrinkage that leaves some lasting visible damage to their breast(s). The best results are achieved in women with small cancers in the upper and outer quadrants of the breast because the symmetry and size of the breast is not as greatly affected with surgery and radiation in this area.

Radiation treatment is generally given on a daily basis for up to six weeks. Some patients find the time and travel commitment that is necessary to be a drawback, although the actual time under treatment is only minutes per session.

It is now clear that for most women, the same degree of local control can be achieved with either mastectomy or WLE plus radiation. Since the cosmetic results obtained with a lumpectomy and radiation are much more acceptable to many patients, women are beginning to choose breast conservation and radiation as their preferred method of local control. This has been the case at our center, where approximately

75 to 80 percent of our patients choose breast conservation and radiation as their local control treatment.

There are several situations in which it is difficult to surgically clear the cancer from the breast with wide local excision and achieve an acceptable cosmetic result. Two obvious situations are a large invasive cancer in a small breast and a cancer that is located centrally beneath the nipple. Chemotherapy can be used in these situations to shrink the cancer prior to surgery, allowing for less tissue removal, lesser scars, and reduced deformity. Italian scientists have pioneered this approach and have successfully "downstaged" the tumor in two-thirds of the women originally rejected as candidates for breast conservation.* After the chemotherapy, this determination was reversed, thereby allowing them to avoid mastectomy. This technique of giving chemotherapy prior to surgery is known as neoadjuvant chemotherapy. (Adjuvant chemotherapy is given to women with a suspected systemic spread of cancer cells after surgery.)

Breast conservation and radiation are also not recommended when there is an extensive amount of ductal cancer in situ (DCIS), either associated with an invasive cancer or purely in its noninvasive form. Because the cancer cells can move along the ducts fairly easily, the cancer involvement can be widespread within the breast. For reasons unknown, these cells are somewhat resistant to radiation. It may be that the cells in the ducts are in a relatively low oxygen environment, and oxygen is necessary for radiation to work. In any event, DCIS cancers associated with extensive intraductal involvement have local recurrence rates after radiation that are as high as 30 percent. An additional consideration is that radiation makes later reconstruction of the breast more difficult because of skin changes. Women who have received radiation and later desire reconstruction often require the tissue transfer–type of reconstruction (discussed later in this chapter).

---

* G. Bonadonna, U. Veronesi, C. Brambilla, et al., "Primary Chemotherapy to Avoid Mastectomy in Tumors with Diameters of 3 cm or More," *Journal of the National Cancer Institute* 82 (1990): 1529–45.

Because of these factors, many women with diffuse or extensive DCIS choose mastectomy as the method of local control. The great paradox is that a woman with a diffuse preinvasive cancer, a cancer that is not a threat to her life, requires a mastectomy.

At our center, half of the women having mastectomies have this significant DCIS type of cancer. The rest choose mastectomies for any number of reasons. Some women are not concerned about breast preservation and do not want the six-week inconvenience of radiation treatments. Others have a fear of radiation or have a collagen vascular disease, as discussed earlier. In spite of all the scientific evidence that mastectomy or lumpectomy and radiation work equally well, there is still a small group of women who are only comfortable with a mastectomy because they want to get rid of the part of their body they feel is diseased. Ultimately, the course of treatment is every woman's personal choice. Once the medical and scientific data have been presented to you and you make your decision, your treatment team should support your choice.

For women who require or choose mastectomy, they should strongly consider reconstruction. Many women reject this option initially because their main focus is survival. Discussing cosmetic reconstruction at the time of the initial surgery may seem self-indulgent and premature to many. But if you are considering a mastectomy, it is important to give reconstruction your serious consideration as well. If reconstruction can be safely done at the time of the mastectomy, the cosmetic result is often superior to that achieved at a later time.

Even if it is necessary to do a delayed reconstruction, it is important for the surgeon to plan ahead, leaving adequate skin and appropriately placed scars that will ultimately result in a better cosmetic result. This will require consulting with a plastic surgeon to discuss reconstruction options. Ideally, the consultation should be done before the mastectomy.

It is not my intention to imply that breast reconstruction is required for optimal living. It is a personal choice. Many women are comfortable with breast removal, and the absence of a breast does not affect their self-image. There are excellent external customized prostheses available for women that desire them.

Clearly, breast reconstruction does not compromise survival and may actually be an important factor in a woman's recovery. The vast majority of women who have reconstruction are pleased with the results.

For the woman who chooses or requires the removal of her breast, breast reconstruction is an alternative to wearing an external prosthesis. Over the years, techniques have been refined so that most women receive excellent cosmetic results with reconstruction, including the creation of a nipple and areola that looks natural.

When breast reconstruction is performed at the time of the mastectomy, it is known as immediate reconstruction. Immediate reconstruction has the following advantages:

1. The need for a separate surgery later is often eliminated.
2. The patient has a newly reconstructed breast immediately after her initial surgery, which, for many women, makes the mastectomy easier to deal with psychologically.
3. The cosmetic result may be better than that with a delayed reconstruction because the plastic surgeons and the cancer surgeons work as a team to achieve the optimal cosmetic and therapeutic outcome. Together, they are able to ensure that there is sufficient skin for a reconstructed breast and an incision that allows for the best cosmetic result.

Immediate reconstruction is most appropriate for women who will not need cytotoxic chemotherapy. Women who require no chemotherapy—those with diffuse DCIS, for example—have the option of having the reconstruction at the same time as the mastectomy surgery. For those women who will require chemotherapy, we suggest delaying reconstruction in the event that there is a problem with healing or infection that would delay the initiation of the chemotherapy.

Delayed reconstruction is appropriate for any woman who may have undergone a previous mastectomy. If you are planning a delayed reconstruction, it is still helpful for you to see a plastic surgeon prior to the mastectomy. Communication between the plastic surgeon and cancer surgeon will often lead to a better cosmetic result no matter how long the reconstruction is delayed.

There are two basic types of breast reconstruction following a mastectomy. The first technique involves the insertion of a device that allows for the creation of a mound giving the appearance of a breast. This "expander" is often replaced by a permanent device followed by the creation of a nipple and areola. An inflatable balloon device is placed behind or on top of the pectoral muscle and sequentially filled with saline (salt water) through an access port that is placed beneath the skin (Figure 2.7). This inflating process takes weeks to several months; then a permanent silicone or saline implant is inserted. In spite of the ongoing debate about silicone implants, I have seen very

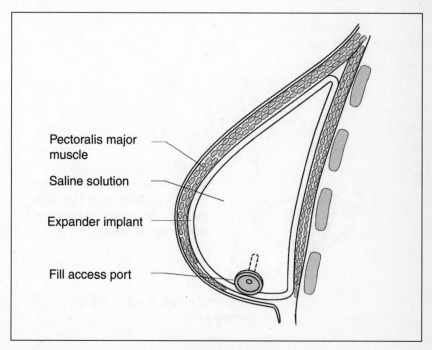

Pectoralis major
muscle

Saline solution

Expander implant

Fill access port

FIGURE 2.7
Breast reconstruction implant

few problems with either the saline or silicone implants. Many women may require minor surgery, such as a lift or reduction of the non-cancerous breast, to give their breasts symmetry and balance. This is often accomplished at the time of the insertion of the permanent implant.

The second major reconstruction technique involves the transfer of tissue from another area of the body to form a new breast (Figure 2.8). This transfer of skin and underlying fat must have a blood supply, which usually comes from an underlying muscle. The blood vessel and its origin muscle are made into a pedicle so the skin and fat can be moved to the chest through a tunnel created by the surgeon beneath the skin's surface. This pedicle of fat with its blood supply is then tailored to form a breast. The sources of tissue are usually from the back

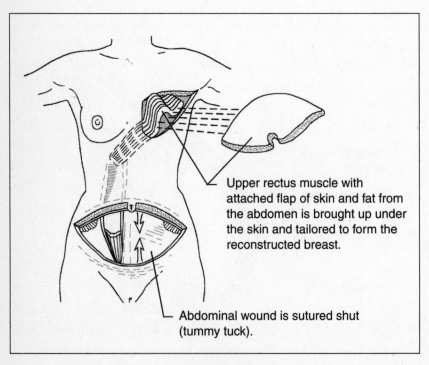

Upper rectus muscle with attached flap of skin and fat from the abdomen is brought up under the skin and tailored to form the reconstructed breast.

Abdominal wound is sutured shut (tummy tuck).

FIGURE 2.8

Breast reconstruction—tissue transfer

(latissimus dorsi transfer) or the abdomen (transfer of rectus abdominal muscle, or TRAM).

This technique, known as tissue transfer surgery, takes many hours and involves wounds in two different areas, at the breast and at the origin muscle site. The muscle and blood vessel with accompanying fat are expendable, and the site of origin heals without any major bodily dysfunction. This surgery has the advantage of incorporating a woman's own tissue, making a foreign device unnecessary. With many women, tissue transfer produces a better result than expander reconstruction, but it requires a much more extensive operation and significantly longer recovery time.

A further modification of the tissue transfer technique involves microsurgery, in which the tissue is completely removed with its blood vessel and reconnected to a new blood vessel in the chest area. This "free transfer" technique allows for less muscle to be removed and no tunneling, which is often required for the abdominal type of surgery.

Some women are not good candidates for tissue transfer because of a lack of fat or previous operations and scars. Also, women who smoke cigarettes have a much higher complication rate for this procedure because of vessel disease.

Recently breast surgeons have developed a technique known as a skin sparing mastectomy that allows for a more normal appearing reconstruction. This technique preserves much of the skin. The breast surgeon removes the breast glandular tissue along with the nipple, leaving a majority of the skin to envelop a saline or silicone implant, or even transfer tissue from another site. The technique requires that the surgeon leave as little underlying breast glandular tissue as possible without compromising the vascular supply to the skin. The small risk of a local recurrence of cancer in the skin flap is acceptable because it should be able to be detected just under the surface by palpation at an early stage. The deep or posterior edge of the resection of breast tissue at the chest wall has an extremely low risk of recurrence because of a natural separation plane known as the pre-pectoral muscle fascia that allows the surgeon to completely remove all the breast tissue in this area (Figure 2.9).

If you are interested in reconstruction, you will want to discuss the various options with your surgeon and ask to see a plastic/reconstruction surgeon in consultation. It is important that both your cancer surgeon and your reconstruction surgeon work well together.

Lobular breast cancer accounts for approximately 15 percent of all breast cancers. It behaves differently from the ductal type. The cell of origin (see Figure 2.3) is the cell at the bud of the terminal duct. This cell, in its normal healthy state, manufactures milk when a woman is lactating.

There is a "premalignant" change in lobular cells in which they divide and fill up the hollow space inside the bud. Initially, we called this lobular cancer in situ (LCIS), thought to be similar to ductal cancer in situ (DCIS). LCIS has no mammographic or physical signs and is always discovered in a breast biopsy that has been taken as a result of other symptoms such as a benign lump. We now know that, unlike DCIS, LCIS does not always result in a progressive cancer. In fact, only 30 to 40 percent of women with LCIS eventually develop an invasive cancer. Invasive cancers are ductal 50 percent of the time or lobular 50 percent of the time. They can appear in the opposite breast as frequently as in the breast where the LCIS was originally found.

So, unlike the situation with DCIS, you cannot remove LCIS and prevent the development of an invasive cancer because LCIS is not the precursor to the ultimate malignancy as it is in DCIS. It is only an indicator that all of the breast tissue is more susceptible to malignant change. The treatment for LCIS is careful surveillance, although some physicians suggest and patients choose preventative, or prophylactic, mastectomies in these cases.

Invasive lobular cancer, also known as infiltrating lobular carcinoma, begins to spread by penetrating the normal breast tissue without actually forming a mass. The mammographic changes can be minimal

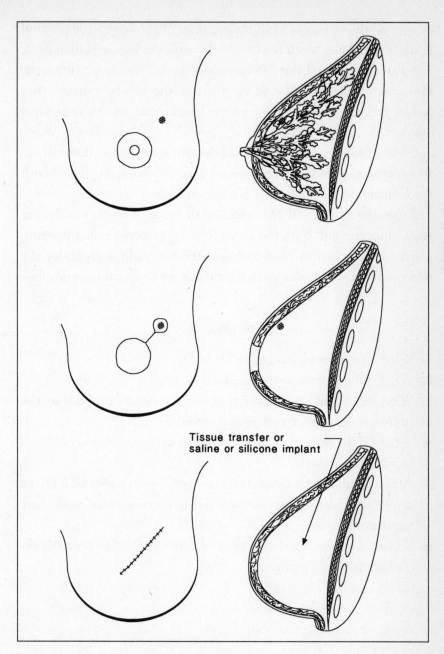

Tissue transfer or
saline or silicone implant

FIGURE 2.9
Skin sparing procedure (mastectomy)

or very subtle, and large areas of involvement can have little physical findings until later, when the extent of the cancer is greater than 2 cm.

Size for size, ductal and lobular cancers have very similar cure rates. However, due to the difficulties in diagnosing lobular cancers, they tend to be larger in size and have more lymph node involvement when discovered.

Some lobular cancers appear like ductal cancer, but without the in situ component. Some breast cancers take on characteristics of both the lobular and the ductal cell in the same tumor.

Regardless of the cell of origin and the type of breast cancer, the goals of local control are the same: to remove surrrounding margins. Local control often involves sampling the regional lymph nodes and removing involved nodes with as little damage to function as possible.

CHECKPOINTS

1. What type of breast cancer do I have?
2. What is the probability of cure for this type?
3. What are the statistical chances of a local recurrence? What are the statistical chances of a systemic recurrence?
4. What are the risks and benefits of breast conservation and radiation versus mastectomy?
5. Am I a candidate for lymph node conservation or removal? If I have my lymph nodes removed, how will this information be used in my treatment plan?
6. If mastectomy is my choice of local control, should I consider reconstruction? If so, when?

3

Systemic Control

In spite of complete and successful local control, breast cancer cells can break off from the primary breast tumor and spread into the blood system prior to complete and successful local control being achieved. Presently, there is no absolutely accurate way of knowing or predicting whether a cancer has spread in the early phases prior to or during diagnosis. However, the earlier we discover the cancer and achieve local control, the less chance there is of its systemic spread to other parts of the body.

After studying the movement of cancer in thousands of women, researchers have now identified certain prognostic factors that allow us to estimate, on a statistical basis, whether cancer cells have spread into the bloodstream. The truth is, however, that you are not a statistic. You are unique on this earth. Either your breast cancer has spread systemically, or it hasn't. We have no absolute way of knowing whether it has spread; all we can do is determine the probability of this happening. We will discuss this topic in depth a little later.

If the cancer has spread, treatment aimed at wiping out these abnormal cells and their potential harm is more successful early in the disease, when they are at their smallest number. This treatment, known as systemic therapy, includes medicines, hormones, and chemicals that are delivered throughout the body to destroy the cancer cells wherever they may be. Unfortunately, these treatments are powerful and have side effects because of their toxicity.

A majority of women with breast cancer do *not* have systemic spread, so systemic therapy does *not* need to be part of their treatment plan. We use the prognostic factors mentioned earlier to help decide the potential need for systemic therapy. Since we are fighting an enemy we are not sure exists, the treatment is known as empiric, or based on practical experience. We measure success over time as the patient's life goes on and there is no sign of relapse.

We know from scientific studies that systemic treatment does work in a percentage of women who take it. In the early 1970s, there were studies done in which women with breast cancer were assigned to two different groups by a "flip of a coin" technique called randomization. One group received chemotherapy, and the other group did not. Over time, there were a significantly higher number of women in the group getting the systemic chemotherapy who did not have their cancers return. In the end, the difference in cure rates between the two groups was between 25 to 35 percent in favor of the treated group.

In the intervening years, new drugs, or known effective drugs in new combinations, have been tested in an attempt to improve the cure rate of women suspected to have systemic spread of cancer. This has been a slow process since each new study takes between four and ten years to produce meaningful information and requires large numbers of women who are willing to enter an investigational treatment program.

Once it was established that systemic therapies improved the cure rate, doctors and scientists added and tested new and promising agents against the best-known therapies. This eliminated the need for a no-treatment randomization control group; the new control group was receiving therapies that were known to work. Today women entering into clinical investigations are getting either "state of the art" treatment or an investigational treatment that may have some advantage.

If you'd like to take part in one of these studies, you need to ask your oncologist whether or not you are eligible for any of the current, ongoing national investigations. For more information on clinical studies, see chapter 12, "Clinical Research Trials."

The most pressing question for you to ask your physicians is, "What is the statistical chance of systemic spread in my case?" If, based on all the current prognostic factors, your doctors arrive at an estimate of less than 10 percent, they probably will not advise chemotherapy since that treatment's increased cure rate of several percentage points probably will not justify the risks it poses to you. However, if your doctors determine there is a 20 to 30 percent risk of systemic spread in your case, it means that systemic treatment statistically improves the cure rate.

Regardless of the statistical chance of spread, the final decision about whether chemotherapy will be part of your program or not is one you must make with your treatment team. Your discussion of this matter should be based not only on statistics but also on your beliefs, intuition, and faith.

The use of systemic therapies to kill microscopic deposits of cells that may have spread through the bloodstream is called adjuvant chemotherapy. Drugs used for this purpose are given by intravenous injection (IV), or infusion into the bloodstream. There are a few that can be absorbed into the body when taken orally.

Most of the drugs used in chemotherapy today were well tested on cancer patients with measurable metastatic disease, for example, breast cancer that has developed into tumors in the lung that can be seen on chest X rays, or tumors in the bone that can be seen on a bone scan. These drugs are known to shrink those kinds of tumors. The next step in the testing of these drugs involved using these already identified active drugs as an adjuvant or preventative therapy for women with primary breast cancer who had only the possibility of microscopic spread. These studies demonstrated that adjuvant chemotherapy resulted in an increased cure rate for women who received it, whether they had confirmed spread or not.

How do the systemic therapies work? Some are hormonelike drugs, the leading example of which is tamoxifen (see chapter 11), that enter the cancer cell and turn it off by interfering with the internal messages coming from the genetic blueprints within the cell. Cancer cells that respond to tamoxifen or to other hormone-type drugs have receptors for hormones on their cell surfaces. This receptor information on your cancer can be found on your pathology report (see chapter 4).

Other systemic therapies involve the use of cytotoxic agents, commonly referred to as chemotherapy. The cytotoxic agents are chemicals that interfere with the replication of rapidly dividing cells at different stages of cell division. There are about a dozen of these agents that can kill breast cancer. Unfortunately, these agents are not specific to cancer cells and can be toxic to normal cells in the body as well. Fortunately, normal cells do not divide as fast as cancer cells, and normal cells have the ability to repair damage rendered by these drugs that is usually lethal to cancer cells.

Newer agents currently under investigation include substances ranging from antibodies to gene products that appear much more targeted and specific to breast cancer cells. This new use of biologically engineered agents promises to be the long-sought-after answer to targeting breast cancer cells specifically and eradicating the disease without compromising normal cells.

As noted earlier, adjuvant systemic therapy kills the microscopic spread of breast cancer cells and has been proven to increase the cure rate. But the chemicals involved in *this* therapy are toxic, and although these toxic effects are temporary, for the most part, they definitely decrease the quality of life while a woman receives the therapy. The likelihood of side effects must be one of the considerations when a woman is making decisions about her treatment. I discuss side effects in great detail in chapter 10.

Patients receive cytotoxic chemotherapy an average of four to six months. The drug tamoxifen is given for three to five years. A number of controlled experimental trials have helped oncologists come up with these ideal durations of therapy, beyond which the benefits diminish.

Who should receive adjuvant systemic therapy is the major question that doctors treating cancer must address. As stated earlier, there is no absolutely accurate test to determine this. Researchers have put tremendous resources and energy into looking for an accurate predictor of microscopic systemic spread, but the perfect test has been elusive. Instead a number of prognostic factors, based on information from the primary cancer and its regional spread to the lymph nodes, are used to determine the best course and length of treatment.

An oncologist can analyze all these factors and determine your statistical risk of relapse. The prognostic factors most frequently used in this analysis are listed here in order of importance, and each one will be explained in turn.

1. Size of the invasive primary cancer
2. Spread of cancer to regional lymph nodes
3. Histologic grade of the cancer (how malignant it is under the microscope)
4. Vascular invasion, the microscopic spread of cancer cells into blood vessels or lymphatic system
5. Analysis of the cancer's DNA for the amount and percentage of cells going through DNA synthesis, also known as ploidy and S phase determination
6. Other factors such as hormone receptors and the presence of increased oncogenes, which are genes or gene fragments that are abnormally overproduced as the result of cancer's presence and may have critical functions affecting variables such as growth rate and drug resistance

This basic knowledge will be critically important for you when you interpret your own pathology report. It will allow you to make your own informed decisions regarding the risks and benefits of systemic therapy.

Size of Primary Cancer

The size of the primary breast cancer can be measured from the thin sections of tissue put on glass slides for the pathologist to interpret. The usual measurements recorded are the largest diameter of the tumor or cancer seen on the slides. The cancer is usually a sphere of millions of cells with supporting structures or framework. We are most concerned about the invasive cancer, not the associated DCIS (noninvasive intraductal component).

Lobular cancer often does not take on a spherical or three-dimensional circular configuration, but spreads in a much more diffuse, erratic fashion. For this reason, measuring lobular cancer is often very difficult. We do the best we can using the pathological specimen, physical exam, and imaging findings from mammograms, X rays, and such.

Regardless of other prognostic factors, cancers less than 9 mm have very little chance of spreading into the bloodstream. Oncologists measure the size of the cancer using a system provided by the American Joint Committee on Cancer. This is called a staging system. The pathologist measures the primary cancer after its removal and gives it a staging number, which is based on the diameter of the three-dimensional tumor.

The categorization of the primary tumor by size is presented in Table 3.1. Examples of tumors of various sizes and stages are provided in Figure 3.1.

Cancer Staging Number	Diameter of Tumor
T1	0–20 mm (0–2 cm)
T1a	0–5 mm (0–.5 cm)
T1b	5–10 mm (.5–1 cm)
T1c	10–20 mm (1–2 cm)
T2	20–50 mm (2–5 cm)
T3	>50mm (>5 cm)

TABLE **3.1**

Categorization of the primary tumor by size

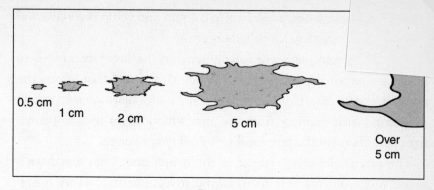

0.5 cm

1 cm

2 cm

5 cm

Over
5 cm

FIGURE 3.1
Tumor size and staging

Cancer in the Lymph Nodes

✳ As we have seen, breast cancer that has spread to regional lymph nodes is a predictor of the cancer's movement into the bloodstream. The more lymph nodes that are involved, the higher the chance that cells have spread to the bloodstream. However, I have followed a number of women who have survived for more than ten years who had many involved lymph nodes. These women had no evidence of systemic spread and were not treated with chemotherapy. Therefore, while lymph node spread is a negative prognostic factor, you should be aware that it is not an absolute predictor of spread.

The following system is used to categorize the lymph node status (N) and is combined with the tumor size (T) system illustrated in Table 3.1.

NO   No involved nodes
N1   Involved node or nodes
N2   Involved nodes that are fixed to one another

You may wonder how many nodes are in your axilla (armpit). There is individual variation, but the average number of nodes is between fifteen and thirty. These nodes are in a chain and go up the axilla and then under the clavicle, or collarbone.

When necessary, surgeons usually remove the lower two levels of nodes and avoid the highest level (level 3), the one that affects the arm (see Figure 2.5). Not removing level 3 nodes helps surgeons avoid interfering with drainage from the arm, which might lead to permanent and often painful arm swelling called lymphedema.

The extent of cancer's spread to the lymph nodes can vary from a small, single, microscopic focus to the involvement of every lymph node that is ultimately removed. The degree of lymph node involvement has important prognostic value. If one considers only the *size* of the invasive cancer combined with *lymph node involvement*, then the chance of systemic spread increases by 10 percent for each 15 mm of size of the primary cancer and 6 percent for each lymph node involved. For example, a woman with a 15 mm (1.5 cm) breast cancer and two involved lymph nodes has a 22 percent chance of systemic spread (10% + 6% + 6% = 22%). Another example: if a woman has a 9 mm tumor and no lymph node involvement, she has less than a 10 percent chance of systemic spread (<10% + 0% = <10%).

Remember that these calculations do not take into account other factors, such as the DNA information and how the cancer looks under the microscope, both of which can also affect your doctor's determination of the risk cancer poses for spreading in your case.

If the oncologist can decide, solely on the basis of the primary tumor size, that a woman will benefit from systemic chemotherapy, it may not be necessary to remove nodes that could contain cancerous cells. However, many women find this concept distressing and ask, "If you don't remove the lymph nodes and by chance they are involved, can the cancer spread to the bloodstream from the nodes themselves?" We do not know the absolute answer to that question, but we think it is *no*.

A number of studies have been done in which women have been put into two randomized groups, one group receiving a lymph node removal and one group not. There is no difference in survival and cure rate between the two groups. Women not receiving a node removal have a slightly increased chance of developing cancerous lymph node(s) at a later time, which would require surgery, but there is no increase in systemic spread. Also, women who get radiation to the lower axilla, which is a fairly standard practice as part of breast radiation, have reduced nodal recurrence. Chemotherapy and tamoxifen also reduce axillary appearance of cancer.

Recent clinical studies and newer technology may make traditional full lymph node dissection and removal unnecessary in most cases. Through the use of a radioactive tracer or a blue dye that is injected into the cancer or the adjacent tissue, the first node receiving lymph node drainage from the cancer can be identified. This node is called the sentinel node or the blue node. Studies indicate that when this node is negative for cancer, there is little chance of finding cancer in any of the other lymph nodes in the axilla.

Doctors use the radioactive tracer as follows: They inject it in and around the cancerous area at the time of the initial cancer surgery. (In cases where the surgeons have removed the cancer in a previous surgery, the doctors inject the radioactive tracer adjacent to the remaining biopsy cavity.) In the operating room, using a portable Geiger counter known as a gamma probe, the surgical team identifies the first draining node and removes it following the removal of the primary cancer. The pathologist then analyzes the node using a technique called frozen sectioning. He freezes the node by using liquid nitrogen and then cuts the tissue into thin slices and views them under the microscope. If he sees no cancer, no further surgery is performed.

The method of using blue dye is very similar but requires the surgeon to inject blue dye that can be visually identified as it is taken up by the lymph system and carried to the first draining lymph node. The lymph node is identified after an incision is made in the lower axilla. It is removed and analyzed as previously described.

Some centers are using both techniques together. It rarely happens that the further analysis of the node, done after additional processing, reveals cancer. When this occurs, you and your doctors may consider further surgery.

I am very enthusiastic about these techniques because today a majority of women diagnosed with early breast cancer will have no lymph node involvement and these techniques can readily identify those women who do not need full axillary lymph node dissections. This will eliminate expense and the small but real risk for arm swelling and nerve damage that can occur as a result of lymph node removal.

In summary, there is some controversy regarding the need for removal of lymph nodes and the method by which this is done. We are clearly in a period of change. Patient risks with node removal include a small possibility of nerve damage and permanent swelling of the arm, while the actual removal of the nodes does not appear to increase the cure rate. Its benefits include providing additional information regarding your prognosis and the need for chemotherapy. You should discuss the topic of lymph node removal with your treatment team and carefully weigh the pros and cons before making any decision.

You should also be aware that there is another staging system that converts the T and N system into clinical stages. You may see reference to this system in your reading or in your reports. The conversion of the T and N system to clinical stages is provided in Table 3.2.

Histologic Appearance of the Cancer

We can tell a lot about the behavior of a cancer by how the cells look under the microscope. As stated before—and I cannot emphasize this enough—breast cancer is a heterogeneous disease, meaning there is not one specific look to all cancer cells. There is, instead, a continuum of malignant change that occurs in cancer cells. A cancer cell can appear as anything from what seems to be a fairly normal duct cell (except that it keeps dividing) to a cell so bizarre that it loses almost all similarity to a normal breast duct cell.

Nodal status (N) and Tumor size (T)	Clinical Stage
T1N0	I
T1N1	IIA
T2N0	IIA
T2N1	IIB
T3N0	IIB
T1N2 or T2N2	IIIA
T3N1	IIIA
T3N2	IIIA
Inflammatory or direct extension into the chest wall	IIIB

TABLE 3.2

Conversion of nodal status (N) and tumor size (T) to clinical stages

Grading this degree of malignancy can be used to predict the chance of cancer cells' spread to the bloodstream. We use a system that looks at three separate features of cancer cells. Called the Bloom Richardson Grading Scale, it is the most commonly used grading system among breast pathologists.

Three aspects of breast cancer cells are evaluated under the microscope:

1. The ability of the cells to form tubular structures
2. The nuclear size, shape, and staining intensity, which is a function of DNA content and its activity
3. The number of cells dividing at a given time, referred to as the mitotic rate

Each of these aspects is given a score of 1, 2, or 3, depending on the degree of malignant change, and a grid can then be formed. A minimal score of 3 and a maximal score of 9 can be achieved with this model. In Table 3.3, the cancer is given a 2 for tubular formation, a 2 for nuclear size, and a 1 for mitotic rate. This results in a total score of 5 out of a possible 9. You will see this written as 5/9.

Bloom Richardson Score	1	2	3
Tubular formulation		X	
Nuclear size		X	
Mitotic rate	X		

TABLE 3.3

Example of Bloom Richardson Grading Scale with a score of 5/9

The Bloom Richardson (BR) scale is further organized into three grades (see Table 3.4). Knowing how to read the BR scale will help you immensely in understanding the nature of your cancer and will be helpful in treatment planning discussions with your oncologist. If we use the example in Table 3.3, the BR score of 5/9 would make this a Grade I tumor.

The BR scale becomes especially important in small breast cancers that measure between 10 and 20 mm (the so-called T1c) and that are lymph node negative (recorded as T1cN0). If one of these cancers has a BR score of 8 or 9, or a Grade III, then the statistical chance of systemic relapse is 20 percent or greater, perhaps justifying consideration of chemotherapy. If it is a Grade I (BR score 3 to 5), then the risk is less than 10 percent, probably not justifying chemotherapy.

Bloom Richardson Score	3–5	6–7	8–9
Grade	I (Low)	II (Intermediate)	III (High)

TABLE 3.4

Bloom Richardson conversion from score to grade

Vascular Invasion of the Cancer

❧ In addition to features scored in the BR scale, the pathologist can look for the presence of cancer in small blood vessels. When such evidence is present, the cancer is more likely to spread into the bloodstream, and chemotherapy should strongly be considered as a treatment option. This feature is often associated with high-grade breast cancers.

High-grade cancer actually has the ability to promote the formation of small blood vessels, a process called neovascularization. The pathologist often recognizes these increased capillaries and blood vessels.

Currently, there is active research under way to identify these blood vessel growth factors. Once these factors have been identified, it may be possible to develop specific inhibitors of neo-vascularization and decrease the chances of systemic spread in breast cancer patients.

DNA Analysis of the Cancer

❧ DNA is the genetic material of chromosomes found in the nucleus of each cell. Each cell in the body has forty-six chromosomes, the diploid number. The only exceptions are reproductive cells (germ cells, including sperm and ovum), which have half the amount, the haploid number. When cells prepare to divide, the chromosomes make copies, line up, and divide—with half the DNA going to each new daughter cell. The cells are exact copies of each other, only smaller. The event is called mitosis. See Figure 3.2.

Cell division in cancer can get very disordered, with more than half of the DNA going to one daughter cell and less than half to the other. The cell with too few chromosomes may lack the essential blueprints to survive, and consequently it dies. The cell with extra DNA has sufficient DNA plus some. When this cell divides, it now gives rise to two daughter cells with more than forty-six chromosomes. Because of this occurrence, the cancer population has extra genetic material that we can measure.

Cancer cells containing the correct amount of DNA are called diploid, while cancer cells with too much or too little DNA are termed aneuploid. Aneuploid cancers have more of a tendency to spread into the bloodstream than diploid cancers.

The method of determining the amount of DNA in a population of cells also gives your pathologist information on the percentage of cells duplicating their DNA material in preparation to divide. This is the percentage of cells in the synthetic phase, or S phase, which tells us how fast a cancer is growing or dividing. Cancers with S phase percentages over 10 percent have more of a chance of spreading into the bloodstream than those with lower S phase percentages.

How important is DNA and S phase compared with size, nodal involvement, and histology? The latter are better predictive factors of systemic spread, but the former are helpful in borderline cases when doctors and patients are deciding whether chemotherapy is necessary.

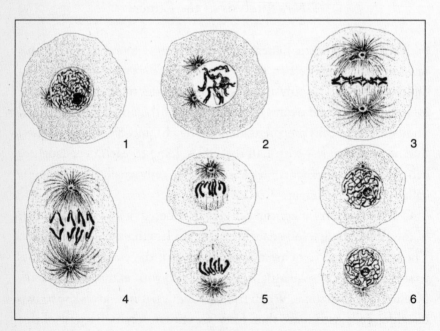

FIGURE 3.2
How cells divide (mitosis)

Other Prognostic Factors

✁ Researchers are searching for "the perfect test" that will predict systemic involvement. Monoclonal antibodies to cancer cells are being developed that, when combined with special stains or radioactive material, may allow them to find small deposits of spread (metastatic cells). Using these techniques, researchers have studied bone marrow from women with early, localized breast cancer (Stages I and II) in order to detect cancer cells. The results, thus far, have been interesting but inconclusive.

Certain breast cancers produce excess genetic material, called oncogenes, that can be measured. You may read or hear about the P53 oncogene or the Her-2/neu oncogene. The Her-2/neu oncogene leads to protein receptors on the cell surface of the cancer cell. There is a direct relationship to the amount of oncogene and the surface protein receptor. An antibody has been developed to the receptor that appears to have therapeutic value (more about this in chapter 9).

Normal breast cells, both ductal and lobular, are under the influence of female hormones, particularly estrogen and progesterone. Researchers discovered a number of years ago that these cells have receptors for estrogen and progesterone on their cell surfaces that can be measured. Breast cancer cells may or may not retain these receptors depending on the degree of malignancy and the number of mutations that have occurred within the cells themselves. Approximately 50 percent of all breast cancers retain these hormone receptors. They are more frequently seen in ductal breast cancers in postmenopausal women and occur in high frequency in lobular cancers.

Because hormone receptors are associated with cancers that are better differentiated, those with a lower BR score, they add no more prognostic information than the histologic grade and thus doctors don't consider them an independent variable. However, they *are* powerful predictors of what the likely response of those cancer cells will be to hormonal treatments.

As you can see, there are complex differences in breast cancers. You will need to meet with your physicians to analyze the characteristics of your breast cancer and weigh the risks versus benefits of using systemic therapy. This can be a very difficult decision. In chapters 9 and 11, we will discuss chemotherapy and tamoxifen in detail so you will have a better understanding of the real and potential risks of whichever treatment you choose.

In the next chapter, we will look at a typical pathology report of a breast cancer surgery. With the information from the present chapter and chapter 2, you will be better able to interpret your own pathology report.

CHECKPOINTS

1. What are the characteristics of my particular cancer (its size, possible spread to the lymph nodes, and the way it looks under the microscope)?
2. What is the statistical risk of my cancer spreading into the bloodstream?
3. Is the cancer influenced by hormones? Does it contain hormone receptors? How might these factors affect the choice of therapy?
4. Is the removal of lymph nodes necessary for planning adjuvant systemic therapy?

4

The Pathology Report

You will want to see your pathology report. In the past, physicians usually felt that it was better for their patients to have limited access to their medical reports. Physicians wanted to interpret the medical jargon because they were concerned that their patients might misunderstand and possibly distort the results they were given. But, today, this thinking has changed among many doctors. The philosophy at our center and at many others is that you have every right to read your pathology report, even if it contains bad news. We want to help you understand the meaning of this information regarding your body so that you can become an integral part of your own healing team.

Our center has worked closely with our breast pathologists to develop and format a report that provides consistent and meaningful information. When we conduct a second opinion, we review a patient's tissue slides along with the original pathology report, which includes a description of the tissue received in the laboratory (called a macroscopic description).

It should be noted that only the original pathologist has the opportunity to view and describe the original piece of tumor. After this description is completed, the tumor is sliced into smaller pieces to make slides for later microscopic evaluation. While subsequent doctors can review the slides, they still must rely on the original description of the tumor itself. It is important for this description to accompany the slides for your second opinion; it is critical to the treatment plan that doctors will draw up and present to you.

See Figure 4.1 below for a sample pathology report of a fifty-eight-year-old woman.

CLINICAL NOTES

Preoperative diagnosis

Right breast cancer

Specimen(s)

A. Right breast tissue

B. Right axillary contents

GROSS DESCRIPTION

A. Received fresh, labeled "right breast mass" is fatty tissue measuring 6 x 5 x 5 cm. Orientation is indicated by double short suture at 6:00, double long at 12:00, and a single long at 9:00. The specimen is inked, medial: blue, lateral: black, superior: red.

Serial sectioning reveals a hard white nodule located centrally measuring 1.9 cm in diameter. It is at least 1 cm from all margins. Representative sections are taken for histologic review. A section from the tumor is sent for hormone receptors and DNA analysis.

B. Received unfixed "right axillary contents" are 62 grams of fibrofatty tissue. There is a suture at one end of the specimen (highest). Nodes are searched for. "B1" lymph nodes farthest away from suture. "B2" central lymph nodes. "B3" lymph nodes closest to the suture.

MICROSCOPIC DESCRIPTION

A. This is an invasive ductal carcinoma. There is abundant tubule formation, moderate nuclear pleomorphism, and rare mitosis. There is no lymphatic involvement seen and no necrosis. There is a small associated intraductal component (5%) of low nuclear

grade with a cribriform pattern. Surrounding tissue shows no associated lobular atypia. The margins are free of involvement.

B. Sections of 11 lymph nodes reveal 1 involved node furthest away
from the suture. This node is partially replaced by metastatic ductal carcinoma and does not extend through the capsule.

FINAL DIAGNOSIS

A. anatomic site: Breast, right, partial mastectomy
   size of specimen: 6 x 5 x 5 cm
   size of tumor: 1.9 cm
   histologic type: invasive ductal, low grade
   histologic grade: 4/9 modified Bloom Richardson
                               scale (BR)
                               1/3 tubule formation
                               2/3 nuclear grade
                               1/3 mitosis
   tumor necrosis: not present
   in situ carcinoma (CIS)   present
   type CIS: ductal, low nuclear grade, cribriform
   percentage: 5%
   EIC (extensive intraductal
   component):   not present
   margins of resection: free of tumor
   nipple involvement: NA
   microcalcifications: none
   background: no hyperplasia or atypia
   ER/PgR: pending
   lymph nodes: 1/11 nodes positive for cancer

FIGURE 4.1

A sample pathology report

The treating oncologist would sit down, go over this pathology report, and apply the information from the report to the woman. Critical
information in addition to this report would be her age, whether or not

she has been on prior hormone replacement therapy, her previous medical history, and so forth.

The pathology report (Figure 4.1) reveals that this fifty-eight-year-old woman has a T1cN1, Stage IIA, breast cancer. As defined previously, this means that the cancer approaches 2 cm in size and that one lymph node is involved. Under the microscope, it is a low-grade breast cancer histologically. In support of this is the DNA data, seen in the prognostic report (Figure 4.2), which shows that the cancer cells have a diploid pattern (amount of DNA equal to a normal breast cell). The number of cells going through S phase is low (replication speed of the tumor cells), consistent with the low mitosis score on the BR scale. The margins are clear. There is only a small amount of in situ cancer. The hormone receptors are both positive.

Reasonable conclusions from this pathology report would be that the woman with this cancer would be an excellent candidate for breast conservation with a low probability for recurrence after radiation. The risk of systemic spread in this particular cancer approaches 20 percent based primarily on the one involved lymph node. Because the patient is postmenopausal, tamoxifen alone or following a regimen of cytotoxic chemotherapy would be a reasonable choice for systemic therapy.

The purpose of this exercise has been to demonstrate how important the information retrieved from the gross and microscopic descriptions of the tumor and the ancillary testing is in developing a treatment plan.

CHECKPOINTS

1. How do I obtain my pathology report? The hospital pathology department or cancer surgeon should be able to provide a copy.
2. Is my pathology report formatted so that I can interpret the information for decision making? If not, will my doctor be available to sit down and explain its contents thoroughly to me?

PROGNOSTIC REPORT
Breast Cancer Prognostic Index

Patient Name: *Example*
Age: DOB: / /

Hospital: *Long Beach Memorial*
Physician: *Link, John*
Hosp./Med. Rec. Number:
Pathology Number:
Account Code: *LBMMC*
Aeron Number:

Prognostic Summary

Good	78	164	1.0		3.8		neg

| | ER | PR | DNA Index | S phase | Her2/neu |

| Poor | |

Prodex Data Values—Frozen Tissue
(see reverse side for interpretation)

Receptor Analysis
Biomechanical

Estrogen: ■ Positive ≥ 10 fmol/mg
___78___ *fmol/mg*   □ Negative

Progesterone: ■ Positive ≥ 10 fmol/mg
___164___ *fmol/mg* □ Negative

DNA Analysis

DNA Index _1.0_ ■ diploid □ aneuploid □ tetraploid
S-Phase   _3.8_ % □ low <8% □ high 8–10%
Comment:

K167 Proliferative Capacity
□ low < 10% staining   □ high ≥ 10% staining
Comment:

EGFR: □ Negative
_____ *fmol/mg* □ Positive ≥ 10 fmol/mg

Her2/neu: ■ Negative
                  □ Positive ≥ 10% staining

Cathespin-D   □ Negative
_____ *pmol/mg* □ Positive ≥ 70 pmol/mg

p53:   □ Negative
                  □ Positive ≥ 10% staining

Comment:

Clinical Information

Tumor site: *Right Breast*

Tumor type: *Infiltrating Ductal Carcinoma*

■ Primary

□ Metastatic

General Comments

FIGURE **4.2**

A sample prognostic report

3. What is the stage of my cancer using the T and N system?
4. Does my cancer contain hormone receptors?
5. What is the statistical chance that my cancer has spread into the bloodstream?
6. Are additional tests indicated?

5

Types of Breast Cancer

The vast majority of breast cancers originate from the lining cells (epithelium) of the ducts or the secretory cells at the terminal ductal lobular unit (Figure 2.2). These malignancies are termed carcinomas. Rare malignancies of the supporting stromal cells occasionally occur and are termed sarcomas. Figure 5.1 shows a pie graph of various types of breast cancer. The malignancies that follow are those originating in the breast.

Ductal Cancer

As previously discussed in chapter 2, ductal cancer has a pre-invasive stage known as ductal carcinoma in situ (chapter 6 is devoted to this). Once the cancer cell penetrates the basement membrane and invades the underlying supportive tissue, it is an *invasive ductal cancer* (IDC). A majority of IDCs have no special characteristics that the pathologist can identify. They vary in their degree of malignancy, and this is graded using the Modified Bloom Richardson Grading Scale (BR Scale) described in chapter 3. About one-half of ductal cancers will have hormone receptors on their cell surfaces and about 20

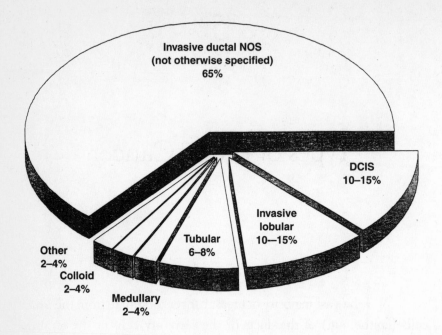

FIGURE 5.1

Distribution of breast cancer subgroups

percent will overexpress the Her-2/neu oncogene. Well over half of all breast cancers will be ductal carcinomas without special characteristics.

These cancers will often lead to a production of a dense fibrotic reaction within the breast tissue that shows on a mammogram as a white stellate structure. Once large enough to be felt, a lump of this origin is quite firm in relation to the surrounding breast tissue. Figure 5.2 is a microscopic photograph of an invasive ductal cancer.

Lobular Cancer

✀ This is often termed "infiltrating" lobular carcinoma (ILC) because the cancer cells infiltrate the supporting tissues in a linear fashion (see Figure 5.3). This pattern of interspersed cords of cancer cells among

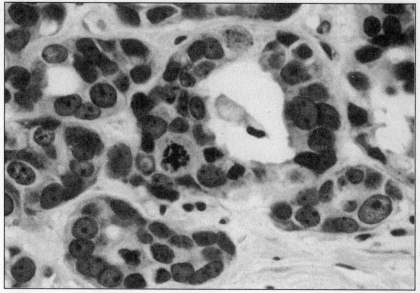

FIGURE 5.2
Invasive ductal carcinoma

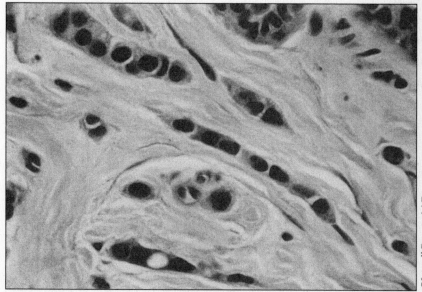

FIGURE 5.3
Invasive lobular carcinoma

normal breast tissue can make both mammographic diagnosis and detection by palpation more difficult.

The association of ILC with a change in the terminal lobular units characterized by atypical lobular cells filling the terminal glandular bud was thought to be the preinvasive phase of ILC. This proliferation of cells was termed lobular carcinoma in situ (LCIS) and was felt to be similar to DCIS in invasive ductal cancer. With more study we learned that LCIS was not necessarily a malignant change and when found by itself in a breast biopsy, it did not go on to give rise to an ILC in most cases. Its presence did, however, lead us to believe that the breast tissue in both breasts was more prone to cancer of both the ductal and lobular types, and this increased risk was two to three times the average woman's risk.

LCIS is a misnomer and does not represent a true carcinoma but a "marker" of increased risk. There has been an attempt by breast cancer specialists to change the term from LCIS to lobular neoplasia. This is in a transition stage now, but ultimately this new term will be used exclusively because it more accurately describes the disease.

ILC accounts for about 15 percent of breast malignancies. It has a similar prognosis and incidence of systemic spread as do the intermediate grade (Grade 2 BR Scale) ductal breast cancers. There is a more aggressive form termed the pleomorphic type that behaves like high-grade ductal cancer.

ILC is hormone receptor positive 80 percent of the time and infrequently overexpresses the Her-2/neu oncogene. Size for size ILC has a similar cure rate as ductal cancer but tends to be discovered at a later stage because of the pattern of growth.

Tubular Cancers

❧ These cancers account for approximately 5 percent of breast cancers. They are of ductal origin and can be thought of as very low grade, well-differentiated carcinomas with a low (Grade I) BR Scale. Under the microscope, the pattern is of somewhat normal appearing ducts (tubules) with mildly enlarged nuclei and no basement membranes. They are usually small (less than 2 cm) and contain hormone receptors. The cure rate is very high with local therapy alone.

Colloid (Mucinous) Cancer

This type of ductal breast cancer accounts for 5 percent or less of breast malignancies. In this type the cancer cell retains the ability to secrete mucin, a liquid material that accumulates within the cells. This type of breast cancer has a good prognosis. It is well differentiated and is not prone to spread into the lymph and blood systems.

Papillary Cancers

This variant of ductal breast cancer is quite rare, and under the microscope the cells form patterns that look like fern fronds. There can be an intraductal or in situ form often involving a larger milk duct. The invasive form is well differentiated and has an excellent prognosis. Because papillary cancers tend to be central in the breast, often behind the nipple and areolar complex, local control without deformity can be difficult.

Inflammatory Breast Cancer

This type of breast cancer involves a high-grade cancer cell of ductal origin that has a high propensity to spread to lymph vessels, especially just beneath the skin or dermis. There often is no mass or lump, but swelling and redness that looks like infection or mastitis—thus the name *inflammatory*. The usual course of treatment before the diagnosis of breast cancer is made is a trial of antibiotics without a response followed by a skin biopsy that reveals cancer cells in the dermal lymph vessels. This type of breast cancer is very aggressive, and surgical re-moval—even mastectomy—will not control it locally.

However, treatment has evolved that has greatly improved the out-look for women with inflammatory breast cancer. Chemotherapy given as the first step often dramatically changes the breast to a normal appearance and then makes local control with surgery and radiation feasible. Women with inflammatory breast cancer require aggressive chemotherapy and I encourage them to look into a number of ongoing clinical trials using dose intensification and newer agents and dosing schedules for this specific type of cancer.

One of the research questions in inflammatory breast cancer is whether women with complete responses to chemotherapy require a mastectomy prior to radiation in order to complete local control. Be-cause this type of breast cancer is quite rare, clinical trials are difficult to conduct and therefore it has been difficult for researchers to obtain meaningful statistical results.

Presently at our centers, if a woman has a complete response with all cancer gone on re-biopsy after chemotherapy, we do not recommend mastectomy but proceed to radiation at that point, usually with further chemotherapy.

Women with inflammatory breast cancer may want to consider inquiring at a major cancer treatment center about possible ongoing clinical trials that they might qualify for.

Cystosarcoma Phylloides

This unusual tumor can be noncancerous or malignant. The dis-tinction, at times, can be difficult for the pathologist to make. Its pre-sentation is usually that of an enlarging mass in the breast of a young woman. Clinically and imaging wise, the lump usually looks and feels like a benign tumor known as a fibroadenoma, a common occurrence in young women. However, these lesions can grow large and grow rapidly, unlike fibroadenomas. Fibroadenomas seldom exceed 2 cm in size. The cell of origin in a cystosarcoma phylloides is probably a supporting stromal cell. When it converts into its malignant form it resembles a sarcoma. It does not spread to lymph nodes, and it does not involve the duct system. The malignant form rarely spreads via cells into the blood system.

Treatment is surgical with a clear surgical margin. Lymph node sampling is not necessary. Women with large tumors, which make breast conservation impossible without major deformity, should consider a skin-sparing type of mastectomy with immediate reconstruction (see Figure 2.9). It has been my experience that the nipple and areola can also be spared in these cases because these tumors do not involve the ducts.

Medullary Cancer

This is a rare type of breast cancer most often seen in younger women. It is dense, cellular, and well circumscribed, which means it is round with a well-demarcated border. Under the microscope it is high grade and looks ominous, but often has lymphocytic immune cells surrounding the border. In spite of its ominous appearance under the microscope, medullary cancer has a much better prognosis than a high-grade ductal cancer of equivalent size. However, this diagnosis is sometimes difficult for the pathologist. For this reason, many pathologists request an outside opinion on the diagnosis because of the possible confusion of medullary cancer with a high-grade ductal cancer with some overlapping features.

Other Types

There are very, very rare malignancies of the breast that originate from the lymph (lymphoma), or from fat (liposarcoma), or from the skin or its glands. These account for less than a fraction of one percent of all malignancies of the breast.

CHECKPOINTS

1. What type of breast cancer do I have?
2. What is the probability of cure for my type of breast cancer?
3. What are the statistical chances of a local recurrence?
4. What are the statistical chances of a systemic recurrence?

6

❧

Ductal Cancer in Situ (DCIS)

This chapter is written specifically for women with ductal cancer in situ (DCIS). If you have invasive breast cancer, you probably will want to skip this chapter for now and move on to chapter 7, "Picking Your Team." Because of the increasing incidence of DCIS, which is about 20 percent of newly diagnosed breast cancer, and the controversies and complexities in management, I felt it was necessary to devote an entire chapter to this topic. As mentioned earlier, the reason for this increase in detecting DCIS is the excellent screening mammography currently being performed at breast screening centers.

As we discussed in chapter 2, DCIS is a ductal cancer that has not penetrated the basement membrane separating the milk duct from the underlying breast tissue, which contains blood and lymph vessels (illustrated in Figure 2.3). If the cancer can be detected at this stage, there is no risk of its spread into the blood or lymphatic systems. This means your risk of dying from breast cancer is essentially zero if it is controlled locally.

Fortunately, DCIS is relatively easy to detect before invasion occurs. It usually appears on a mammogram as a speckling of calcifications that has a characteristic appearance to the mammographer (see Figure 6.1). The calcifications are dead cancer cells that have "petrified" or calcified

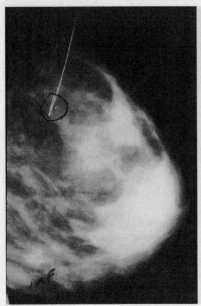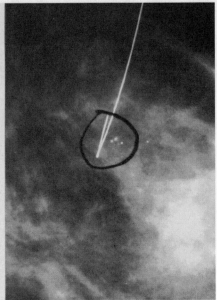

Small cluster of calcification   Magnified view with hook and wire
(low-grade DCIS)

FIGURE **6.1**
Mammogram with calcifications

inside the ducts. These "flecks" of calcium have nothing to do with your calcium intake.

Like invasive breast cancer, DCIS is a heterogeneous disease. All DCIS has the common feature of not penetrating the basement membrane of the breast. According to the medical literature, a majority of these cancers will become invasive if left untreated or undiscovered. The cell that becomes cancerous can vary in its aggressiveness and growth rates.

Some forms of DCIS are low grade and very slow growing. Under the microscope, the cells are fairly small and resemble normal small ductal cells. The nuclei in these cells are relatively small, without extra chromosomal material, and there is little evidence of cell division. This form of DCIS is often associated with mammographic calcifications that have a powdery appearance on the mammogram. Under the microscope, there is not much in the way of necrosis, or dead cellular material, in the center of the ducts (see Figure 6.2). Because of the absence of necrotic material, known as comedo necrosis, this type of DCIS has been termed noncomedo.

At the other end of the spectrum of DCIS is the high-grade form, which is fast growing, has large nuclei full of extra chromosomal material, and gives rise to prominent areas of central duct necrosis with characteristic calcifications that look like branching tree limbs (see Figure 6.3).

If this type of DCIS is allowed to grow and become invasive, it is potentially very dangerous because of its rapid growth rate. This type of DCIS, often termed comedo, has necrotic material that oozes out when the duct is cut by the surgeon or pathologist.

There are intermediate forms of DCIS that fall between the two ends of the spectrum. Since this is an area of breast cancer we have

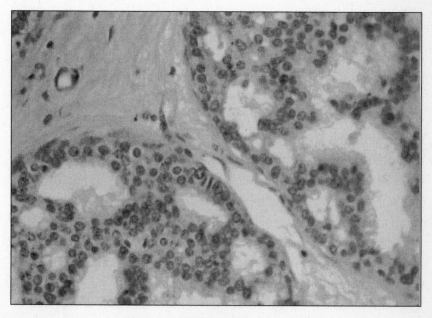

FIGURE 6.2
Small cell without necrosis

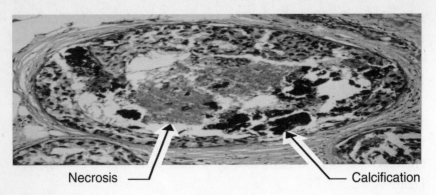

Necrosis ———/ ———— Calcification

FIGURE **6.3**
DCIS: Large cell with necrosis

only two decades of experience with, we are just beginning to understand the nature of DCIS and how to manage it.

The challenge of treating DCIS is removing it completely from your breast. The treatment of DCIS has primarily been surgical. The involved ducts must be removed with a clear surrounding margin of normal breast tissue. The margin of uninvolved breast tissue is important in preventing recurrence from cancer cells that could be left behind if an involved duct is transected during the biopsy. Ideally, the breast surgeon looks to remove tissue and leave a 10 mm clear margin with normal ducts between the edge of the biopsy and the cancerous duct. This can be difficult if the area of DCIS involvement is larger. The extra 10 mm margin that the surgeon must remove in these cases can increase the size of the biopsy substantially and leave the patient with a large divot or a much smaller breast. The mammographer can greatly assist the surgeon in planning the best surgical approach possible. Since there is no palpable lump with DCIS, the mammographer must assist the surgeon by placing markers, usually in the form of a wire hook, where the cancer appears in the breast tissue. Then the surgeon knows exactly what portion of tissue must be removed.

Breast surgeons learned from early experience that if the area of DCIS was small and they cleared wide margins in an excisional biopsy, it would not recur in most women. For larger areas of involvement, it was often impossible for doctors to clear the margins adequately to prevent recurrence yet leave the breast with an acceptable size and symmetry. In these latter cases, most women chose simple mastectomy, often with immediate reconstruction, with a cure rate of essentially 100 percent.

Recently, clinical trials have demonstrated that radiation in addition to surgery reduces the recurrence rates when the cancer's involvement is larger and the margins are close. Radiation, however, is not as effective when DCIS is large and high grade.

Complex questions concerning DCIS include whether DCIS can be treated with wide local excision alone or WLE with radiation. We have as our standard the simple mastectomy (removing the nipple and underlying breast tissue without removing the draining lymph nodes), which is 100 percent effective. The question for the patient with DCIS is whether to do a mastectomy with a 100 percent cure rate or WLE with or without radiation yielding better cosmetic results but lower cure rates.

If there is careful follow-up after wide local excision or wide local excision with radiation, on average, only 10 percent of women with DCIS will experience a recurrence. These recurrences can be found early and necessitate more surgery, most often a mastectomy. The cancer discovered in a situation like this is still usually preinvasive and not life threatening. If the initial treatment includes radiation, the type of reconstruction that can be performed if a mastectomy and reconstruction are required later is limited. Once radiation is used, an expander type of reconstruction is more difficult to do. Doctors must consider each case carefully to determine if breast conservation therapy is possible. The surgeon and mammographer must work together to come to a conclusion, and they will depend on the pathologist for information on invasion, cell type, and margins to do so.

Recently, Drs. Melvin Silverstein, Michael Lagios, and Pamela Craig at the Van Nuys Breast Center in Southern California developed a system for assessing DCIS and its treatment. The goal with this system (or any of the others that may come along) is to achieve an acceptable local control rate, preventing the risk of invasive recurrence with an acceptable cosmetic result. The Van Nuys group looked at their extensive experience with DCIS and concluded that the three critical factors in predicting local recurrence in DCIS patients treated with less than mastectomy were (1) size of breast tissue with DCIS calcifications on mammogram, (2) cell type as determined on biopsy, and (3) extent of clear margins at surgery. They developed a scoring index based on these three factors, giving a score of 1, 2, or 3 in each of the categories, not unlike the Bloom Richardson Grading Scale discussed earlier. Table 6.1 shows the Van Nuys Prognostic Index (VNPI) for DCIS. What makes this scoring system useful is that it appears to be able to predict local recurrence rates using excisional biopsy with or without radiation. These predictions are based exclusively on retrospective analysis; still, the system is an admirable attempt to put some order into this very difficult area of breast cancer management.

If a cancer's score is 3 or 4 on the Van Nuys Index, then local control can be achieved with excision alone. If the score is 5, 6, or 7, then radiation is necessary to bring the local control rate up to the 90 percent range. With a score of 8 or 9, even the addition of radiation does not give acceptable local control rates, so mastectomy is the recommended treatment.

Index	1	2	3
Size	0–14 mm	15–40 mm	> 40 mm
Cell type and necrosis	Low and intermediate nuclear grade without necrosis	Intermediate nuclear grade with necrosis	High nuclear grade with necrosis
Extent of clear margins	> 10 mm	1–9 mm	< 1 mm

TABLE 6.1

Van Nuys Prognostic Index for grading DCIS

Although DCIS is a preinvasive, early breast cancer, it sometimes calls for a mastectomy. Occasionally, DCIS is discovered just as the cancer cell has developed the ability to penetrate the basement membrane, and this early invasion (often called a microinvasion) is reported by the pathologist. When we see a microinvasion, we consider it the same as pure DCIS as long as the amount of invasion is small. Once the invasion involves several millimeters, we consider this a small invasive breast cancer and it crosses the line from the preinvasive stage into a T1a lesion. Like DCIS, T1a breast cancers have a cure rate that approaches 100 percent.

CHECKPOINTS

1. Is my surgeon working closely with the mammographer in planning the best surgical procedure to remove the DCIS with adequate margins?
2. Is the pathologist reporting the type of DCIS, the presence or absence of necrosis, and a measurement of the cancer-free margin?
3. What will be the downside of adding radiation? What will be the improvement in local control?

7

·······

❦

Picking Your Team

The diagnosis and treatment of breast cancer have changed dramatically in the last twenty years. Twenty years ago, a majority of women who had a palpable lump went directly into surgery. Often, the operation was a mastectomy, and that was the full extent of their treatment. Researchers were beginning to explore the role of adjuvant chemotherapy, and radiation was a new course of treatment utilized by a few brave women.

Today, the majority of breast cancers are discovered by mammography. These cancers are small, often too small to be felt, and surgeons rely on radiologists to find or localize them with a hook wire or some injected blue dye. As you can see, the technology has changed dramatically, and we have entered a new era of breast cancer diagnosis and therapy. Because of the many elements that come into play in cancer diagnosis and treatment, coordination is required among a team of physicians: surgeon, radiologist, pathologist, radiation oncologist, plastic surgeon, and medical oncologist.

Ideally, a woman with a newly diagnosed breast cancer connects with a key physician who takes charge of developing a treatment plan with her and then coordinates its implementation. These team members can work at a single institution or be drawn from a wider geographic area, and any of the cancer specialists can act as the coordinating physician. In our institution, it is usually the medical oncologist who coordinates the flow of information and treatment for a patient, but many of our surgeons and radiation oncologists take on this pivotal role as well.

I hope you will find a cancer specialist you can communicate comfortably with and who will address your concerns. However, there are medical systems in which it may be difficult for the patient to connect with one physician who will act as her coordinating team leader. If this describes your situation, don't despair. This manual will give you adequate information to help you get the treatment you need and be your own team leader. It is possible to go through this process without a physician to spearhead your treatment plan and still get "state of the art" care.

The overall treatment plan revolves around two critical decisions. One deals with local control and the second with the need for systemic adjuvant therapy. Often you and your doctors cannot decide upon the issue of systemic therapy until all the information is available from your surgical procedure.

Since the diagnosis and the treatment of breast cancer are done primarily in an outpatient setting, you may well travel to various locations for different aspects of your treatment. In our community, some women come to our center for the definitive surgery and then have radiation at a facility closer to their home. If you require various therapies, you may want to consider doing something similar in order to make your treatment appointments as convenient as possible.

From your first decision about who to contact for a second opinion all the way through your many follow-up exams after your treatment is completed, communication is the key. You, the patient, must establish a relationship with a physician that will enable you to develop an overall treatment plan and have it flow as smoothly as possible. You might also want to get to know the nurses well. Nurse specialists often play very important roles by coordinating and facilitating the communication process between you and your doctors.

At our center, one of the key tools used in coordinating a woman's care is the treatment planning conference. This conference is a meeting of the team members to discuss each woman's case and to develop a coordinated treatment plan based on the patient's individual situation. The conference allows each of the team members to review a common history, the radiological breast images, the pathology report, and the pathology slides.

The patient is usually excluded from the treatment planning conference in order to allow an honest and candid exchange between the team members to take place. Ideas may be offered and challenged as the treatment plan is forged. This process could become inhibited if the patient herself were present, not to mention the confusion and anxiety this discussion of options could provoke in the woman, who needs a concise, clear-cut direction.

Even though you do not attend the conference, you should be apprised of the process and the conclusions of the discussion. Some centers actually have formal minutes or written conclusions that they provide to patients. Other centers arrange for the conclusions to be verbally presented to you by the team member coordinating your care. Usually, the discussion and recommendations made at the pretreatment planning conference are shared with you by the physician who presented your case to the group.

The treatment planning conference is extremely important in coordinating care. Each of the potentially treating physicians can, in one setting, agree on an overall treatment plan and their particular contribution to that plan. This united approach also guarantees that the doctors line up the sequencing of the different therapies correctly and in the manner that is most beneficial to the overall well-being of the patient.

In our breast center, this conference also allows us to identify women eligible for special research tests and protocols sponsored by the government or other research groups. This is an important aspect of our program that offers our patients "state of the art" care and promotes medical advancement.

Besides benefiting the individual woman with breast cancer, the nature of the conference itself promotes education and understanding on the part of the various physicians involved. It also allows younger physicians and physicians in training to attend and witness the treatment planning of a number of women, which would otherwise take them years to accomplish in their own individual practices. In addition, women diagnosed in the future stand to benefit greatly from the shared pool of information that these conferences provide medical professionals in general.

CHECKPOINTS

1. Has a sequential long-term plan been developed before beginning any treatment (i.e., surgical operation, radiation therapy, chemotherapy)?
2. Do I have a key physician or nurse specialist whom I can call on for problems or questions? Is he/she willing to communicate with other physicians on my team as my treatment plan evolves?
3. Am I eligible for any research studies by the National Cancer Institute (NCI) or National Surgical Adjuvant Breast and Bowel Project (NSABP) that might benefit me?

8

·······

❧

Radiation

Radiation is a local treatment administered by specialized physicians known as radiation oncologists. It is given with a large machine called a linear accelerator that converts radioactive particles into a high-energy radiation beam that is used to treat a specific, well-defined area of your body. Radiation affects cells in the area of the tissue beneath the directed beam of radioactive particles, and dividing cells are affected more by radiation than resting cells. Cancer cells are, therefore, more affected than healthy cells, but both cancer cells and normal cells are damaged by radiation. However, normal cells have a greater ability than cancer cells to repair themselves following radiation exposure. Radiation puts cancer cells into a cell death cycle at the time of the next scheduled division. This death cycle is called apoptosis.

Many of our patients often do not clearly understand the role radiation plays in the overall treatment plan. For instance, they wonder why radiation is necessary if a breast cancer has been removed by a wide local excision (WLE) with clear margins. In spite of local removal, about 30 percent of women will have a relapse without radiation, whereas 5 percent or less will relapse with radiation. Pathologists often have difficulty determining if there is a clear margin of normal tissue surrounding the cancer, given the difficulty of measuring the presence of minuscule amounts of cancer cells. Also, it is well known that there may be "skip" areas between the main tumor and small hard-to-detect satellite cancer nodules in the immediate vicinity. Therefore, in spite of clear margins, tumor cells may be resting on the other side of the biopsy margins. Cells may have traveled through the breast duct system and come to rest outside of the biopsy site as well. Radiation is important because it has a good chance of destroying those random cancer cells.

Radiation to the chest surface is sometimes also recommended following mastectomy if the cancer extended to or through the surgical margins or if several lymph nodes are involved with cancer. The addition of radiation in these situations reduces the incidence of local recurrence considerably.

Is radiation always necessary? If we could pick the 60 to 70 percent of women who would not have a local recurrence, then we could avoid radiation in the majority of cases.

Unfortunately, this is not so easy to do. If the cancer is small, with a large clear margin of uninvolved tissue, and if there is no local lymphatic involvement or extensive DCIS, then one might consider observation alone and no radiation, especially if the woman's breasts are very fatty. As a woman ages, the ratio of fat tissue to glandular tissue increases. It is quite normal for the female breast to contain significant amounts of fat, which is not necessarily related to obesity. In fact, thin women can have breasts that contain a large percentage of fat. Fat cells are beneficial in the breasts in that they provide an excellent background for the radiologist to pick up a small cancer or early recurrence on a mammogram. Therefore the fat content of your breasts may be a factor in considering your need for radiation therapy and one you should discuss with your doctors.

Recent studies also indicate that a woman's age may be an important contributing factor for risk of local recurrence if radiation is not done. Dr. Umberto Veronesi, a world renowned breast surgeon from Italy, reported a study in which women received wide local excision with clear surgical margins for small T1 breast cancers (<20 mm). Each woman was then randomly assigned to either postoperative radiation or no radiation. Women over the age of sixty had a less than 5 percent recurrence rate without the radiation! Younger women had a higher local recurrence rate without radiation for reasons that are not clear. These findings have led the Radiation Treatment Oncology Group in the United States to begin a study currently under way that involves women over the age of seventy with T1 breast cancers being treated without radiation. The results of that study might further reduce the use of radiation on older women with breast cancer—we'll see.

The typical course of radiation is daily treatment for twenty-five to thirty sessions. There is good reason to give such extended, prolonged treatment. A long string of short, individual treatments causes less damage to normal tissues, allowing them to repair completely, while increasing the progressive lethal damage to cancer cells.

Receiving radiation treatments involves several steps. First, you will have a consultation with the radiation oncologist, who will explain the risks and benefits of the treatment to you in detail. If radiation is to be part of your treatment, the next step is an expanded planning session, called a simulation session, which can take several hours. Simulation is done using computer modeling to calculate the exact area of treatment and dosage of radiation you should receive. Once the radiation oncologists determine the area of treatment, they will mark the parameters of the treatment field on your body so that every time you have a treatment, the exact same area will be treated. Some facilities use a felt pen to designate the area; others use a small permanent tattoo about the size of a small beauty mark. All of this will be discussed and reviewed with you at the simulation session, prior to beginning any treatment.

Once the actual administration of radiation begins, the treatments are given by a highly trained technician. Your actual daily treatment time ranges from seconds to several minutes. Most women will see their radiation oncologist once a week for monitoring, but remember that your physician is always available for any special problems that may arise from the daily treatment. Don't hesitate to ask to see the doctor with any questions or concerns you may have.

If the margins around the cancer have been cleared surgically and the purpose of the radiation is to eradicate any microscopic cells that may have been left behind, twenty-five to thirty treatments with the linear accelerator are usually adequate to achieve this goal. However, if your team has some question in your case about margin involvement or if there is some component of in situ breast cancer, they may decide to give an extra amount of radiation, called a boost, to the tumor area.

There are several methods of giving boosts. The most common involves the linear accelerator and consists of five to ten additional radiation treatments to the local surgical area. Some centers have the equipment available to use a different type of radioactive particle called an electron. These electrons deliver high-energy radiation to the surgical area in a treatment known as an electron beam boost. The boost is administered externally over five to ten sessions in a very similar manner to the way radiation is given with the linear accelerator.

An alternative method of boosting is the implantation of small seeds of radioactive material, called iridium, into the surgical area. These seeds remain in the breast for forty-eight to seventy-two hours. Your surgeon implants these during a short surgical procedure; however, with the advent of the electron beam method of boosting, doctors are choosing to use these implants less frequently because of the hospitalization required, the expense, and patient discomfort. Now, very similar boosting results can be achieved using the external methods.

There are side effects from radiation to the breast. It is usual to have some skin changes, such as redness and some inflammation that usually fades over time. Ninety percent of women have an excellent cosmetic result after healing occurs. Ten percent have some added fibrous tissue, shrinkage of the breast, and reduced skin elasticity and sensitivity. There are treatments you may use on your own skin to help facilitate healing and reduce the long-term effects of radiation.

These skin side effects are important when considering reconstruction.

The majority of women who have reconstruction following radiation therapy will require the tissue transfer type of surgery called a TRAM flap because of the decreased skin elasticity and pliancy caused by the radiation.

As for other side effects, radiation does pose several. However, with modern techniques, the radiation beam does not penetrate deeply into the body and thereby avoids the lung and heart. The ribs get some exposure and may be tender for a year or longer as a result. You may experience temporary fatigue and a mild depression of the white and red blood cell counts. Many women notice mild to moderate decreases in their energy levels during their course of treatment, but there is no associated hair loss or major problems with nausea that often accompany chemotherapy.

When a woman needs both chemotherapy and radiation, chemotherapy is usually given first. This is because several of the chemotherapy agents raise the toxicity of the radiation and can cause increased skin changes if given simultaneously. Also, if the treatments were to be given at the same time, the bone marrow would suffer a greater impact, resulting in lower white blood cell counts, which can leave a patient more vulnerable to infection.

Many women express concern regarding radiation treatment and its ability to cause other cancers later in life. In order to understand the danger of this possibility, you should know the risks involved with a number of sources and types of radiation that human beings are exposed to. Some are environmental, such as solar radiation, and are considered "natural," while others are man-made, such as those resulting from X rays and imaging. It is true that in large doses, radiation is carcinogenic and can cause genetic mutation. This is often the result of partial injury to a cell that recovers and goes on to divide and pass on defects to offspring chromosomes.

These defects do not result from therapeutic radiation thanks to the P53 gene. This remarkable gene is in each cell and appears to protect the cell from most of these mutations. Fortunately, if a cell is injured, the P53 gene prevents further cell division until repairs are made. It is amazing that the body has such self-healing potential.

A number of studies have been conducted to determine if there is an increased risk of a second cancer in patients treated with therapeutic radiation. Retrospective studies have looked at women receiving primary radiation for the treatment of breast cancer and the incidence of a second breast cancer and other types of malignancy. The bottom line is that there is a very *slight* increased risk of a second cancer as the result of radiation treatment. Women who have had radiation therapy have approximately a 1 percent chance of getting a second breast cancer from the treatment itself, compared with women who have not received radiation in the treatment of their breast cancer. Age seems to be a factor, and the highest risk occurs for women exposed to radiation at a young age. The risk for women over age forty appears to be negligible, but not zero.

CHECKPOINTS

1. Do I need radiation?
2. What side effects should I expect, and when will they occur?
3. How long will my treatment last?
4. How can I best care for my skin in and around the radiated area?
5. What are my chances of getting another cancer later in life as a result of the radiation treatment?

9

Chemotherapy

Traditionally, a cancer diagnosis that called for chemotherapy provoked more distress and fear in many women than the need for either surgery or radiation. In the early days of chemotherapy, administration techniques and dosages were far from optimal. At that time, these drugs were primarily used by oncologists as a last-ditch effort to treat incurable cancers with little regard for the patient's quality of life. It is little wonder chemotherapy has such a bad name.

Fortunately, things have changed dramatically. Today, we have well-researched dosages and administration routines as well as effective supportive medications to minimize the side effects of chemotherapy, making the entire process easier to bear. However, while there have been great strides made, I do not want to understate the power of chemotherapy. This is a very strong toxic class of medications and should not be thought of as simple or without risk.

Chemotherapy administered to women with localized breast cancer is given to kill *possible* microscopic cancer cells that may have reached the systemic circulation. Clearly, many women are willing to undergo moderate temporary toxic effects to substantially increase their chance of cure. Chemotherapy increases the cure rate of breast cancer by approximately 33 percent when there is micrometastatic disease present.

Breast cancer cells are quite sensitive to chemotherapy drugs. The drugs are poisonous to all cells and interfere with the cells' ability to reproduce but are particularly threatening to cancer cells. That is because the more malignant a cancer is, the more rapidly it divides. It is during this process of cell division that the chemotherapy can destroy the cancer cells. Also, the smaller the total number of cancer cells, the better chance the chemotherapy has of killing all of them. Theoretically this is true because single cells or small clusters of cancer cells have plenty of nutrients and oxygen, and divide more rapidly than larger cancerous masses, which have fewer resources to draw from. When cancer cell division slows, it has a chance to develop drug resistance.

Different classes of drugs affect different aspects of cell replication and can be used in combination with each other. This means that drugs may work sequentially. The selection of drugs and their combinations are based on the results of a number of clinical trials involving thousands of women that have taken place over the past twenty years. Initially, a new drug is tested on women who have advanced breast cancer. If there is a high response rate or remission rate, then the drug is tested on women with a high probability of microscopic metastatic disease. It usually takes three to seven years to obtain results for this testing process.

Unfortunately, there are no good ways to speed up the test procedure process using animal models or testing the drugs on a cancer outside of the body. The technique of removing cancer cells from a primary tumor and testing them in a culture with various drug combinations and concentrations, as is done with bacteria and antibiotics, makes good theoretical sense, but it is technically difficult and still needs to be refined to produce accurate results. I am hopeful that, in time, researchers will be capable of testing the effectiveness of new drugs on cancer outside the body, selecting medications that work for a particular cancer and eliminating those that do not.

This type of testing was studied for more than ten years. Oncologists were initially very enthusiastic, but the early studies showed an inconsistent correlation between the cells' response to drugs in the lab (in vitro) and their actual response in the body (in vivo). As a result, this method of testing was largely abandoned. I feel that move was premature since the in vitro method was very good at predicting what drugs or classes of drugs did *not* work at achievable concentrations in the body. I thought those benefits outweighed the fact that testing drugs on cancers outside the body had less predictive value regarding which drugs would go on to work at lower concentrations. These studies involved mainly those patients with advanced metastatic disease that was measurable and could serve as the source of the tumor cells. It is possible that micrometastatic breast cancer cells behave differently than the primary cancer.

The proof of whether this testing is of value in micrometastatic breast cancer is almost impossible to obtain presently, since we do not have a highly predictable test for micrometastatic disease. Fortunately, most breast cancers do respond to the major classes of drugs. About 20 percent of the drugs tested against the primary tumor show resistance or inability to kill the cancer cells. When enough cancer is available, we can do these tests, or assays, at one of several available commercial labs.

If we can avoid exposing a woman to a toxic drug that has no chance of working, I believe we should do so. In vitro testing must be done on tissue that is newly removed from the body, so your surgeon must agree to the test and plan ahead to preserve a sample of the tumor. The other issue with this testing has been whether insurance companies will pay for it. Interestingly, when presented with the current data, most insurance companies have agreed to pay for tests like these, but often a doctor and patient must submit a letter of appeal to them before they will agree to cover the expense.

Classes of Chemotherapy Drugs

✻ Chemotherapeutic drugs used to kill breast cancers are classified as follows:

1. *Alkylators*. This is a group of drugs that affect cancer cells like radiation. Cyclophosphamide (Cytoxan) is the most commonly used agent. It is usually given intravenously (IV) but can also be administered orally on a daily basis. The IV form does not usually cause hair loss, but the oral form may. This is a very effective drug and is part of almost every regime used for adjuvant therapy.

2. *Antimetabolites*. These are drugs that act as "false" building blocks and are incorporated into the DNA. When the cell gets ready to divide, a defect occurs that causes the cell to die. The drugs 5-fluorouracil, commonly referred to as 5-FU, and methotrexate are antimetabolites in this category used in breast cancer treatment. 5-FU is a fluoropyrimidine carbamate class drug. It is a false building block for the nucleic acids that are part of the genetic structure in the nucleus of the cell. A new fluoropyrimidine has recently been developed known as capecitabine (the brand name is Xeloda). This drug can be taken orally and requires an intracellular enzyme to convert it to its active form. Breast cancer cells contain more of this enzyme than normal cells, which gives capecitabine a selective advantage in killing cancer cells over normal cells. Capecitabine is presently going through the testing process and is not used in the adjuvant setting at present but may be available in the future. Methotrexate inhibits an enzyme that is important in providing a building block for DNA. The vitamin folic acid can overcome the block, so this vitamin (usually found in the B-vitamins) should not be used while a woman is on methotrexate.

3. *Antibiotics*. These are different from the antibiotics used for treating infection. They are potent inhibitors of DNA replication. The most commonly used drug of this class in breast cancer is doxorubicin (Adriamycin). Adriamycin is extremely active with breast cancer and is usually combined with Cytoxan. A sister drug called mitoxantrone (Novantrone) is less frequently used. In Canada and parts of Europe, another drug very similar to Adriamycin, known as epirubicin, has replaced Adriamycin for

the treatment of breast cancer. Epirubicin appears to have better tolerance and will shortly be available in the United States. I suspect it will rapidly replace Adriamycin in most regimens. Mitomycin, another drug in this class, is active with breast cancer but is not usually used in adjuvant regimes.

4. *Antimitotic agents.* When cells divide, the chromosomes line up and migrate to opposite poles of the nucleus of the cell. The apparatus for the process is called the spindle. Certain drugs inhibit this step of cell division (or mitosis of the cell) and cause the inability of cells to migrate. Vincristine (Oncovin) is an example of a drug that interferes with this process, as is a new drug called vinorelbine (Navelbine).

5. *Antimicrotubule agents.* The taxanes, paclitaxel (Taxol) and docetaxel (Taxotere), are unique agents that originated from the Pacific yew tree. They are very potent in killing breast cancer cells. In a short span of several years these agents went from discovery to rapid testing in several cancer types, including breast cancer. Because of their great ability to kill breast cancer cells and a relatively low toxicity to normal cells, they are now part of many regimens for women who have a significant risk of micrometastatic disease.

6. *Heavy Metals.* Cisplatin (Platinol) is a heavy metal used to kill cancer cells. Its effectiveness as a cancer fighter was discovered in the late 1970s when scientists were trying to pass electrical currents through petri dishes of bacterial colonies to determine if the electronic activity inhibited bacterial growth. Interestingly, the bacteria around the platinum electrodes died rapidly. From this observation, it was discovered that platinum leaked into the tissue media and was responsible for killing the bacteria. This led to further investigations that demonstrated that platinum was a potent inhibitor of cell division and an excellent anticancer drug. Initially, it was used to treat testicular cancer with spectacular success. Most recently, it has been used in ovarian and

breast cancer treatment with similar results. It has good activity and can be used in high doses with moderate toxicity.

One of the present issues and questions being addressed in clinical trials is whether drugs should be used together (combination chemotherapy) or if they should be used singularly in sequence (sequential chemotherapy). If drugs are combined and share common toxicity such as affecting the bone marrow, often the dosage must be reduced, perhaps reducing the effectiveness. Some drugs in combination may be synergistic, meaning the combining of the two enhances the killing effect over what would be achieved by giving the two drugs alone in sequence.

Based on the successful trial results in the treatment of Hodgkin's disease, breast cancer chemotherapy was traditionally given in combination. Early results did demonstrate a combination of drugs were better than one single agent. As new evidence emerges regarding the presence of synergy and drug toxicity from interactions, regimens may contain combined drugs as well as sequential drugs.

The other major issue for medical oncologists treating breast cancer with chemotherapy is dose intensity. The higher the dosage given in a fixed time period, the greater the potential toxicity and risk to the woman. Most often this is bone marrow toxicity with a suppression of bone marrow stem cells leading to decreased white blood cell production, putting the woman at increased risk of infection. Recent evidence suggests that a certain dose intensity must be given to achieve the maximum cancer cell kill, but exceeding this threshold only increases risk without further benefit.

We now have a number of drugs that kill breast cancer cells, and there are new agents in the pipeline. Progress has been made in how to optimally administer these agents, and there are supportive therapies that prevent and aid in a woman's recovery from toxic effects as well.

Several combinations of drugs have evolved and have been commonly used to treat women for possible micrometastatic disease. The standard has been one of two combinations: cyclophosphamide, methotrexate, and 5-FU (CMF); and Adriamycin and cyclophosphamide with or without 5-FU (AC and FAC). With recent evidence that a taxane increases the disease-free survival rate over AC alone in women with breast cancer that involves regional lymph nodes, most oncologists are treating these women with a combination of AC, followed by a taxane.

The new agent, trastuzumab (whose brand name is Herceptin), an antibody to the Her-2/neu protein receptor on the cancer cell surface, has been shown to enhance the chemotherapy effect in women with Stage IV breast cancer (breast cancer that has metastasized to a distant site: i.e., bones, lungs, or liver). Trastuzumab (Herceptin) is presently undergoing testing for the use in women with localized breast cancer that demonstrates an overexpression of the Her-2/neu oncogene. The first trials will involve women with node-positive disease. If your cancer falls into this category and overexpresses Her-2/neu, ask your oncologist if you are elibible to participate. We have much to learn about how to use this new exciting therapy.

Side Effects of Chemotherapy

Many women are uneasy with the idea of enduring "chemotherapy." This is totally understandable. The chemicals make women who still feel well, feel sick. These agents (medicines) *do work*, however, and when used in appropriate situations, they may increase the cure rate of breast cancer by 30 percent or more. The end may indeed justify the means. Until research produces a systemic therapy that is more specific, we will continue to use chemotherapy. Therefore, it is important for you to educate yourself about chemotherapy and its side effects before making a decision on whether to incorporate it in your treatment plan.

A majority of the chemotherapeutic drugs affect all dividing cells in the body. This includes both benign and malignant cells. If a woman has microscopic systemic breast cancer, these cancer cells will be dividing and be more sensitive to chemotherapy than most normal cells. Some of the body's normal cells that also divide on a regular basis are the bone marrow blood-producing cells and the lining cells of the gastrointestinal tract. For this reason, these normal cells are also sensitive to chemotherapeutic drugs.

Of all the side effects of chemotherapy, bone marrow toxicity is the most serious. The bone marrow is the production site of white and red blood cells. A majority of women being treated with chemotherapy for breast cancer will experience a drop in their white blood cell count, usually seven to fourteen days after a treatment. Therefore, while on chemotherapy, it is extremely important for you to be on the alert for an infection, which is one of the first signs of bone marrow suppression. The most obvious symptom of an infection will be a fever.

It is important to alert your physician at the first signs of infection and receive antibiotic therapy. Some protocols routinely put women on antibiotics the second week after each chemotherapy treatment as a preventative measure against infection. There are genetically engineered bone marrow stimulants such as Neupogen and Epogen available for women who develop severe depression of their white or red blood counts, respectively. Fortunately, the toxicity to the bone marrow from chemotherapy is temporary and reversible. If an infection occurs, however, it is potentially very serious and must be treated to avoid life-threatening complications.

Also sensitive are the cells that line the gastrointestinal tract from the mouth to the anus, which the body manufactures and replaces every few days. Some of the chemotherapy drugs can interrupt this production of cells, causing small ulcers. This is unusual in breast cancer treatment, but you should be aware of the possibility. The mouth and rectal areas are the most vulnerable, so you should pay attention to their condition while receiving chemotherapy. If you should notice weak spots, there are local treatments for mouth sores and anal fissures that your oncologist can prescribe for you.

The most common side effects of chemotherapy used to be nausea and vomiting, primarily during the week immediately following treatment. The main cause of nausea is a massive release of substances called histamines, which are stored in the cells lining the gastrointestinal tract. Newer drugs can now prevent the release of histamines. Thanks to the discovery and use of proper support medications, the nausea and vomiting accompanying chemotherapy has been reduced and is much less of a problem than it used to be. The incidence of these side effects varies depending on the drugs used and the intensity of dosage. Although it may be hard for you to believe, some women experience no such chemotherapy side effects at all today.

For many women, hair loss is a very distressing side effect of a few of the breast cancer drugs. Some of the agents such as doxorubicin (Adriamycin), paclitaxel (Taxol), and docetaxel (Taxotere) can cause uniform temporary alopecia, hair loss, especially from the scalp. Other drugs cause only a thinning of the hair. Many of the breast cancer regimes have Adriamycin, and some of the newer ones have Taxol or Taxotere, so you should anticipate temporary hair loss with chemotherapy.

I think it is helpful to understand the mechanism of hair loss associated with these drugs so you realize its true temporary quality. Drugs like Taxol, Taxotere, and Adriamycin interfere with protein production. The cell at the base of the hair follicle makes protein every day, which results in normal hair growth (see Figure 9.1). On the day of chemotherapy administration, the protein that the cell produces is faulty, which makes the hair brittle at that point. This brittle point is protected under the scalp for approximately three weeks, but once it gets to the surface the hair breaks off easily. While hair loss is not easy to cope with for many women, remember that it is only temporary and the hair will soon return. In chapter 10, "Management of Side Effects," I discuss strategies that may help you through this difficult experience.

There are some additional side effects with chemotherapy that are not often mentioned but that you should be aware of. These drugs can often affect nerve endings and lead to a mild neuropathy, which is manifested by mild numbness of the fingers and toes, and a change in

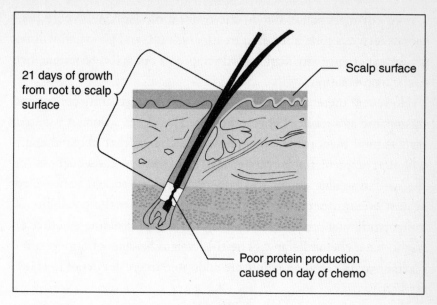

FIGURE 9.1
Hair follicle

taste that many women characterize as being bland, muted, or metal-lic. In addition, some women complain of subtle changes in cognitive function and memory, which are always temporary but can last for the entire course of the therapy. Some patients have referred to this side ef-fect as *chemonesia*, and I have seen several graphic examples of it. One I remember, in particular, was experienced by a woman who had re-cently learned English as a second language. During her treatment she suddenly regressed and struggled with communication, only to have it return completely after the chemotherapy had ended.

The bone marrow toxicity, hair loss, and other side effects are for the most part acute and reversible. For women who have functioning ovaries, however, chemotherapy may have some permanent effects. Chemotherapy drugs affect the production of hormones from the ovary. If a woman is in her midthirties to early forties and her ovaries are fully producing estrogen and progesterone, then chemotherapy may interrupt the production of these two hormones and put her into a transient menopause. Often, the ovaries' production of these hormones recovers fully after drug treatments end, and a woman will no longer experience any menopausal symptoms but go on to resume her cyclic menstruation.

However, there are a few women who will go into permanent menopause as a result of chemotherapy. The closer a woman is to her own natural menopause, the greater the chance that chemotherapy will start it prematurely. Menopause has negative consequences for the cardiovascular system and bone density that should be weighed against breast cancer risks. My own opinion is that the possibility of a premature menopause is not a major factor in deciding whether or not to have chemotherapy. (The risks versus benefits of hormone replacement after ovarian failure are addressed in greater detail in chapter 17.)

Because side effects can be debilitating, many women want to know if they can continue to work while on adjuvant chemotherapy. The answer varies depending on the regime used and the stress and demands of your particular job. Each woman should determine what she is comfortable with as treatment gets under way. Many of the chemotherapy schedules call for the drugs to be administered every two to three weeks. Usually, patients suffer the worst responses in the first few days after each administration. At our center, we often give the chemotherapy on a Friday, and many of our patients have recovered sufficiently by Monday or Tuesday to return to their usual activities. We have observed that good hydration during the first seventy-two hours following chemotherapy administration is important to a rapid and symptom free recovery. If nausea and vomiting occur, this may lead to decreased fluid intake and mild dehydration. This probably leads to increased concentrations of drug by-products as well as cell breakdown products in the bloodstream, thereby increasing kidney function to eliminate them. With any signs of early dehydration we will intervene with intravenous fluids. We have observed that this makes a tremendous difference in recovery. Whether you decide to continue working or not, I suggest that during the several months of chemotherapy you plan to take it easy. Reduce as much of the stress in your life as you can. Engage your loved ones, friends, and extended support system to help you, especially during the periods when you are down and not feeling well.

Bone Marrow or Stem Cell Rescue

With the success in the late 1980s and early 1990s of adjuvant chemotherapy to prevent micrometastatic recurrence, investigators began testing very high doses of chemotherapy in conjunction with bone marrow rescue. It was well known that high doses of chemotherapy often cause severe depression of the bone marrow. But researchers found that by obtaining bone marrow from the patient before the chemotherapy and storing it, they could give her very high doses of chemotherapy and then give her back her own bone marrow. She was, in a sense, "rescued" from the bone marrow depression and recovered more quickly. The hypothesis was that the very high doses of chemotherapy would overcome drug resistance and would kill the few remaining cells that were able to withstand conventional dosages of chemotherapy. Initially, these trials appeared to be very successful on women with metastatic disease.

The women who received the high-dose therapy were first given conventional chemotherapy, usually Adriamycin and cyclophosphamide (AC). If there was a good response to regular dose therapy, they then were given high-dose therapy with a bone marrow transplant (BMT). Women who did not respond to regular dose therapy were not subjected to the toxicity and expense of the high-dose therapy followed by a BMT because of poor results among this group. This was early in the experience of this procedure.

It turned out that the women who received the high-dose therapy with BMT were a highly selected group, and the high complete response rates that were reported did not include the women who were not allowed to receive the therapy due to a poor initial response.

Because of early initial success using BMT in women with metastatic disease, women with a very high probability of relapse were given the high-dose therapy with BMT. Stem cell reinfusion or rescue has since replaced BMT. These women with high-risk, localized breast cancers with more than ten lymph nodes involved, or those with large cancers greater than 5 cm, or others with the rare type of breast cancer called inflammatory breast cancer were then studied. Recently, scientists' reports have clearly demonstrated that high-dose chemotherapy with BMT for women with early metastatic disease prolongs remission. However, the data are somewhat disappointing because the bone marrow rescue does not appear to be curative. The results for women with locally advanced disease and with heavy lymph node involvement look more promising at this point, with a majority of these women remaining in remission at the four- to five-year mark without receiving any further chemotherapy or treatment. These encouraging results led to several randomized trials comparing high-dose chemotherapy with BMT to moderate dose chemotherapy with growth factor support. The purpose was to prove that high-dose therapy with BMT was truly better treatment and to determine if the encouraging nonrandomized initial results were possibly due to selection bias. Selection bias means that the oncologists possibly gave the high-dose therapy with BMT to women whose cancers had characteristics that made them more likely to respond, compared to the historical comparison group.

The results of these several trials have recently been reported at the American Society of Clinical Oncology (ASCO) in May of 1999. At this point, there is no demonstration of a clear advantage to the high-dose therapy with BMT over moderate dose therapy. It should be noted that these trials were begun prior to the availability of the taxanes, which, if combined with the moderate dose regimen, theoretically should further improve the results. I will discuss clinical research in more detail in chapter 12.

High-dose chemotherapy with BMT is very expensive, costing approximately $100,000, and it is quite toxic for the patient. Early on there were a number of treatment deaths, but as centers became more experienced, the death rate fell below 5 percent. There was also controversy regarding whether the therapy was investigational and who should be responsible for paying the bill. There were several highly publicized lawsuits involving women who were denied approval by their insurance companies.

Now that we have more objective data to present to women regarding this procedure, women can make informed decisions with their physician and treatment teams. I feel the evidence at this point demonstrates no major advantage for using high-dose therapy with BMT outside the research setting, and it is certainly more expensive and toxic.

It should be noted that for women at high risk of systemic relapse (large cancers with involved lymph nodes or inflammatory breast cancer; see chapter 5), fairly intense chemotherapy can be given safely in an outpatient setting, i.e., an infusion center at your doctor's office. These regimens often utilize growth factors such as filgrastim (Neupogen), which stimulate bone marrow recovery and lower the risk of infection. Also, with newer agents such as Taxol, Taxotere, and Herceptin, the outlook is much better for women with these types of breast cancer.

Chemotherapy Selection

If your risk of microscopic systemic disease is sufficient to justify systemic adjuvant therapy, how does the oncologist select the type, number, intensity, and sequencing of the drugs for you? Presently, there are ongoing research trials testing all of these things. You may ask your oncologist if you are eligible to receive treatment as part of a trial study. These trials, which are often randomized, usually provide "state of the art" therapy even if you must be assigned to a control group, called a specific treatment arm.

Theoretically, each chemotherapy treatment, of whatever mix of drugs your oncologist chooses, will kill a fixed percentage of the cancer cells. The surviving cells have either resistance, which is usually not the case, or were not vulnerable because the timing of the drug doses didn't coincide with the vulnerable stage of the cell's cycle. Figure 9.2 is a schematic graph of what occurs during chemotherapy. Let's assume that there are 100,000 cells that have escaped the destructive effects of chemotherapy. This figure illustrates a greater than 90 percent kill per treatment, which is realistic. As you can see, there is some cancer re-growth between chemotherapy cycles. It is important not to allow too much time between cycles, otherwise the cancer will recover to its prechemotherapy force; however, a rest period between drug dosages is necessary for the body's bone marrow to recover its strength.

The more intense the chemotherapy, the greater its effect on the bone marrow. The intensity of the chemotherapy regimen is based on

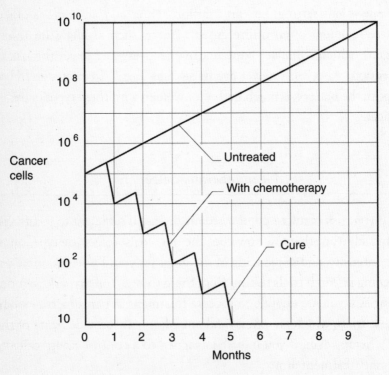

FIGURE **9.2**

Cancer cell kills using adjuvant chemotherapy

the clinical trials testing safety and tolerance of the drugs. The dose limiting toxicity with a majority of the regimens is bone marrow suppression. In the past, oncologists checked the woman's blood before each chemotherapy cycle and modified the dosage based on the white cell count. Today, the bone marrow tolerance is monitored by obtaining a white blood count about ten days after the administration of chemotherapy. Oncologists must balance the risks of possible infection and bleeding of bone marrow suppression against the benefit of increased cancer cell kill from increasing the dosages of chemotherapy. Modifications of dosage or the addition of bone marrow stimulants is based on the results of this postchemotherapy white cell count.

The most standard chemotherapy regimen for node-negative breast cancer is a combination of cyclophosphamide, methotrexate, and 5-fluorouracil (CMF). The drugs are given intravenously (IV) at three-week intervals. Another way your team may give CMF is to administer the cyclophosphamide orally for fourteen days along with IV methotrexate and 5-fluorouracil on day one and day eight. This regimen is repeated every twenty-eight days. (See Table 9.1.)

Each session of chemotherapy lasts between thirty minutes and an hour, and the administration of the drugs is carefully monitored by a registered nurse who is experienced with possible drug interactions and potential side effects. Appropriate nursing care for patients is vital to ensure safety and proper administration of these potent chemotherapy agents.

Most studies indicate the use of Adriamycin offers little advantage over the standard CMF, and it has some increased toxicity. However, there are data that suggest Adriamycin may be more effective in women whose cancer overexpresses the Her-2/neu (Erb-B-2) oncogene. Prior to this Her-2/neu observation, oncologists often recommended Adriamycin in young women with high-grade or node-positive cancer. If you fall into one of these two categories, you might want to ask your oncologist about the benefits of Adriamycin.

Epirubicin is a drug very similar to Adriamycin and has been used in Europe and Canada for a number of years. Recently this drug has been approved for use in the United States by the FDA. At this time there

Drug	Dosage	Method of Administration	Frequency
Regimen 1			
Cyclophosphamide	600 mg/m^2		
Methotrexate	40 mg/m^2	IV	Repeated every 3 weeks
Fluorouracil	600 mg/m^2		
Regimen 2			
Cyclophosphamide	150 mg	oral	Every day for 14 days
Methotrexate	40 mg/m^2 day 1 and day 8	IV	Repeated every 28 days
5-fluorouracil	600 mg/m^2 day 1 and day 8	IV	

TABLE **9.1**

Two chemotherapy regimens using CMF

Drug	Dosage	Method of Administration	Frequency
Regimen 1			
Adriamycin	60 mg/m^2	IV	Every 3 weeks for 4 cycles
Cyclophosphamide	600 mg/m^2		
Regimen 2			
5-fluorouracil	500 mg/m^2	IV	Every 3 weeks for 6 cycles
Adriamycin	50 mg/m^2		
Cyclophosphamide	500 mg/m^2		

TABLE **9.2**

Two chemotherapy regimens using Adriamycin
in combination with other drugs

is no evidence that it is more effective in killing breast cancer than Adriamycin; however, there is a suggestion that it may be better tolerated. It is unclear to me at this point whether epirubicin will replace Adriamycin in the United States. I believe this will depend on future studies that compare the two drugs for effectivenes, toxicity, and cost.

Adriamycin is combined with cyclophosphamide alone or with cyclophosphamide and 5-fluorouracil. (See Table 9.2.)

The taxanes, both Taxol and Taxotere, are very active chemotherapy agents against breast cancer. Clinical trials have demonstrated an increased disease-free survival if given to women with positive lymph nodes.* A taxane is usually given following an Adriamycin containing regimen. The standard has been to give either Taxol or Taxotere every three weeks for a total of four treatments (see Table 9.3); however, other dose schedules are being investigated.

Drug	Dosage	Method of Administration	Frequency
Adriamycin	60 mg/m²	IV	Q 3 weeks x 4
AND			
Cyclophosphamide	600 mg/m²	IV	Q 3 weeks x 4

Drug	Dosage	Method of Administration	Frequency
Taxol	175 mg/m²	IV	Q 3 weeks x 4
OR			
Taxotere	100 mg/m²	IV	Q 3 weeks x 4

TABLE 9.3

Taxane containing chemotherapy

---

*I. C. Henderson, D. Berry, G. Demetri, et al., "Improved Disease-Free (DFS) and Overall Survival (OS) . . . ," *Proceedings of the American Society of Clinical Oncology,* no. 17 (1998): 101a, Abstract 390A.

Preoperative or Neoadjuvant Chemotherapy

In chapter 2, I briefly discussed the use of preoperative (also termed neoadjuvant) chemotherapy. This type of treatment has been utilized to treat women with large (almost always larger than 2 cm), palpable breast cancers.

The use of chemotherapy prior to surgical removal of the cancer has a number of real and theoretical advantages:

1. It shrinks the size of the cancer and allows for easier removal with a better cosmetic result. The Italians demonstrated this and reported that a majority of women who would have required a mastectomy due to the size of their cancer could be treated with breast conservation surgery after preoperative chemotherapy. Multiple studies show less than 10 percent of cancers will grow during chemotherapy, and more than 50 percent will completely regress, based on palpation.

2. It allows for earlier administration of chemotherapy. Women do not have to wait for surgery and healing to begin treatment for possible micrometastatic cancer cells.

3. The cancer may be much less virulent and have less angiogenesis after preoperative chemotherapy, making surgery safer with less risk of spreading cells. This is theoretical and unproven to date, but frequently at the time of surgery there is little viable cancer present. If there is, it is of a lower grade than the original cancer seen at the time of the diagnostic needle biopsy.

4. Women who have good responses to the preoperative chemotherapy have a much better cure rate compared to those women with little or no response. For the women who have palpable remaining cancer, we often will do drug resistance and sensitivity testing on the tissue to determine if some type of alternative or backup chemotherapy agent might be effective.

A possible disadvantage of preoperative chemotherapy is that the extent of lymph node involvement may not be accurately determined.

Previously, this was an important consideration for possible candidacy for high-dose chemotherapy with BMT. However, with the efficacy of this procedure in question, the number of involved lymph nodes may not be as important. I am a strong proponent of the use of preoperative chemotherapy in the appropriate situation. It does require a team approach. The breast surgeon must be willing to postpone surgery, and often the cancer must be mapped or tagged with small, needle-inserted radio-opaque seeds so that the area of cancer can be surgically retrieved if the tumor disappears altogether, which is often the case.

When you are considering the use of systemic therapy, the following questions are key for your oncologist:

CHECKPOINTS

1. What is the risk of systemic spread of my cancer?
2. What is the benefit of cytotoxic chemotherapy? How much will it increase my chance of cure?
3. What is the optimal regimen of drugs to be used? What is available to me to reduce the side effects?
4. Am I a candidate for dose intensification? If so, would I qualify for an investigational protocol and who will pay for it?
5. Does my cancer overexpress the Her-2/neu oncogene? If so, am I a candidate for a trastuzumab (Herceptin) protocol?
6. Am I a candidate for preoperative chemotherapy?

10

Management of Side Effects
Quality-of-Life Issues

With a diagnosis of cancer, your first consideration and priority is survival. Once you and your doctors have developed a plan to optimize survival, you begin to consider how the treatment will alter your life. Recently, there has been significant progress not only in the treatment of breast cancer, but also in the control of the unfavorable side effects of treatment.

Each woman will experience breast cancer and its treatment differently. You will find that physical, emotional, and spiritual aspects all play a role in how you react. The extent of your treatment's side effects depends on the intensity and the amounts of adjuvant therapy you will have as well as your individual life experience and your underlying well-being.

When diagnosed with breast cancer, a majority of women have no symptoms. We often hear women comment on how strange it is to feel physically normal and now know there is a cancer in their body. However, once treatment begins, most women will feel literally "diseased," not from cancer but from the treatment itself. Except for the physical scars, a majority, if not all, of the discomfort and physical changes from the treatment are temporary. We have already discussed the side effects of chemotherapy in considerable detail in the preceding chapter. The purpose of this chapter is to better acquaint you with some other common side effects of cancer treatment so you can work to minimize their effects on and disruptiveness to your life as much as possible. Once you have worked together to develop a treatment plan, your physicians can provide you with assessments of the potential side effects and recovery time you most likely will experience in relation to your specific family responsibilities and career.

Recovery from Surgery

❧ The standard surgical option for the local control of breast cancer involves removing breast tissue. The underlying chest muscles, pectoralis major and pectoralis minor, are no longer removed as they were in the not-too-distant past. This great advance has significantly reduced the pain and recovery time following surgery, but, more important, women are spared the long-term disability of having the muscles removed.

If you have a lumpectomy without the lymph node dissection, you will most likely have surgery and go home the same day. Recovery from surgery will take longer if you must undergo the removal of lymph nodes from the axilla. With their removal the lymph flow from the breast is partially interrupted, and, to minimize a buildup of fluid, many surgeons will place a soft rubber tube in the wound to drain the lymph temporarily, usually for three days to a week. Your length of stay in the hospital for lumpectomy and lymph node removal or mastectomy with lymph node removal is usually one to two days.

The drain from the lymph nodes empties into a closed rubber expandable vessel about the size of a handball. You will usually empty the vessel daily and record the amount of fluid or lymph you dispose of. After several days, the amount of fluid usually decreases rapidly, at which time the surgeon removes the drain. Some surgeons choose not to put in a drain, and if fluid builds up adjacent to the armpit wound, they drain it by inserting a needle and aspirating the liquid.

If you have any lymph nodes removed, most surgeons request that you move the involved arm as little as possible for the first few days following your surgery to allow the edges of tissue to heal and to keep lymph flow to a minimum. Once the drain is out and the wound is healing, you must begin progressive and gentle exercise of your arm to increase the range of its motion in order to prevent permanent limitations from scarring. Some surgeons instruct their patients on exercises, while others refer them to physical therapists who have "post-lymphadenectomy" exercise regimes. (A lymphadenectomy is the surgical removal of lymph nodes.) It is important for you to discuss with your surgeon which option will be best for you.

Following the lymph node surgery, many women will have numbness in the armpit because of the cutting of the nerves in the area. Sensations often return over several months when the nerves grow back. However, a small percentage of women will have permanent numbness here. For those who experience this lack of feeling, it is important to be particularly careful shaving underarm hair. I advise patients who have lost feeling here to use an electric razor.

With the lymph node surgery, a small percentage of patients develop a clotted vein running down the inner side of the upper arm that feels like a thin cord and can restrict arm movement. If this happens in your case, it is important to use heat treatments and do stretching exercises so you eventually have a full return of movement.

Side Effects of Radiation

Radiation effects on your tissues are cumulative. In other words, there is a buildup of the effects of radiation to your body over time. The usual course of radiation, as discussed earlier, is approximately twenty-five to thirty treatments. You will probably see only a few noticeable changes during the first ten sessions or so, but then redness and mild swelling of the skin often appear around the irradiated area. The technologists and staff will be watching for any unusual skin reactions and will recommend appropriate remedies to you as they are needed. There are creams and lotions that can help ease the discomfort of these side effects.

Most women will have a darkening of the radiated area that looks like a suntan. In time, as the skin heals, this usually lightens and disappears. Women have a variety of skin responses to radiation, just as people have various skin responses to sun exposure. My own observation has been that light-skinned women tend to have more of a visible skin reaction to radiation than those with dark skin.

If you have radiation, your underlying ribs can be tender to external pressure for months to several years following your treatment. Although rare, it is possible that a minor trauma can cause a rib fracture because of the weakness in your bones following radiation. But no special precautions need to be taken.

Many women complain of fatigue during radiation. This can be difficult to measure for the woman as well as for the physician. If you require chemotherapy at the same time as the radiation, your weariness can be significant. You should, therefore, just be aware that your energy will be greatly diminished during your treatment and try to plan your activities accordingly.

Most women will have slight skin edema, or swelling, following radiation. The easiest way to see this is at the areola, which is usually "crinkled"; with the swelling your areola will appear quite smooth. Nipple sensation and erectile ability generally remain normal.

Radiation can cause the breast being treated to shrink slightly. If a woman gains significant weight after radiation, it is not uncommon for the nonradiated breast to enlarge more than the one that received radiation. Also, if a woman becomes pregnant after breast radiation, the radiated breast will usually not enlarge and produce milk to the extent that the nonradiated breast will. Most of our patients who have elected to breast-feed following radiation have found that the radiated breast cannot produce a sufficient amount of milk but the nonradiated breast functions normally.

Side Effects of Chemotherapy

❧ As discussed in chapter 9, chemotherapy affects all rapidly dividing cells; although it destroys irregular cancer cells, normal cells recover completely after the treatment is completed. During chemotherapy, you may experience side effects, which you need to be prepared for and contend with.

Your nutrition during chemotherapy is extremely important because you need to provide your body with vital "building blocks" for repairing the damage done to normal cells by the chemotherapy. You must have lots of protein, which contains essential amino acids, and small amounts of fat or oil to ensure that your cells are getting all the essential fatty acids they require. Antioxidant vitamins, which I will discuss at length in chapter 13, are also important in tissue repair and protection from both radiation and chemotherapy damage.

Chemotherapy and Menopause

Chemotherapy also affects the endocrine function of the ovaries in premenopausal women. The ovaries are the body's major producers of estrogen and progesterone, and they create these hormones in a cyclic pattern in response to trigger hormones secreted by the pituitary gland. At some point in a woman's late forties or early fifties, the ovaries no longer produce these hormones and she goes into menopause. The process of the ovaries shutting down their hormone production takes several months to a year or so to happen. This gradual decrease in estrogen and progesterone may cause a variety of symptoms, including the cessation of menstrual periods, hot flashes or flushing, and vaginal dryness. Chemotherapy may accelerate menopause. This means that at the very same time a woman is handling a breast cancer diagnosis, she often must deal with the changes and possible uncomfortable effects associated with menopause. This is also true for the postmenopausal woman on hormone replacement therapy (HRT) who suddenly must stop her hormone replacement treatment because of the diagnosis of breast cancer.

The relationship of breast cancer and estrogen is complex and controversial and should be considered individually in each woman's case. The standard treatment for a newly diagnosed breast cancer patient is to stop HRT. In the past, women with breast cancer were not encouraged to resume or begin to take HRT ever. This practice has changed, and treatment today is based on each woman's individual situation. You must consider the risks and benefits of HRT in relation to your specific case and discuss them with your physician(s).

Chemotherapy in the younger woman and the withdrawal of HRT in the postmenopausal patient can often produce symptoms of menopause that can be distressing and even disabling. This is an area where Eastern medicine can be of great benefit. Certain herbs used for many years by Eastern medical practitioners contain estrogenlike substances that are called phytoestrogens. Some of these herbs relieve symptoms without stimulating breast cancer cells. The following herbs have been found to be helpful: oil of evening primrose, gotu kola, and black cohosh root.

You can obtain these herbs at most health food stores. My experience has been that a majority of women suffering from menopausal symptoms are helped to some degree by one or more of these substances. Some of my patients have been helped quite dramatically. You should discuss dosage and duration of these supplements with your doctor, since they can change depending on your needs and circumstances. In general, the unit doses range from between 250 and 500 mg, and maximum benefit is usually achieved with less than 1,000 mg.

Many women have also found that by making dietary adjustments, they have fewer hot flashes. Soy and soy products contain an estrogenlike substance known as genistein. It is 1/100,000 as strong as estrogen produced by the ovary (estradiol), but it does have the ability to alleviate hot flashes to varying degrees in many women. I will discuss the benefits of soy and other dietary changes to breast cancer patients in chapter 13.

For years, belladonna, an ancient drug derived from a plant of the same name, has been used to control hot flashes. Physicians commonly prescribe belladonna in combination with ergotamine and phenobarbital in a preparation known as Bellergal. Because of the strength of the substances it contains, I tend to prescribe Bellergal only when herbs are not effective and hot flashes are severe enough to lead to sleep deprivation and irritability.

If herbs and Bellergal are ineffective, I often then resort to the use of low-dose progesterone. The safety of low-dose progesterone in women with breast cancer has not been extensively studied, but preliminary data appear to suggest its safety. Many oncologists use low-dose progesterone with tamoxifen, which appears to help reduce hot flashes and prevent uterine lining or endometrial growth. Today many women are also using a natural progesterone product for these symptoms that is made from either yams or soy and that can be administered in the form of a cream. This usually requires a prescription and must be obtained from pharmacies that specialize in custom compounding. (Figure 10.1 summarizes the sequential management of menopausal symptoms in women with breast cancer.)

Many women experience vaginal dryness as a result of estrogen deficiency. There are a number of excellent vaginal moisturizers that are nonhormonal and nonpetroleum based. Estrogen vaginal cream provides an excellent remedy, but the estrogen is absorbed systemically, which usually is contraindicated. The thinner the vaginal membranes, the more estrogen is absorbed, allowing substantial amounts to enter the body. New products are becoming available in the form of slow-releasing estrogen vaginal inserts that provide minimal amounts of estrogen into the body. These help ease the discomfort of dryness but don't provide so much estrogen as to stimulate growth in cancer cells and interfere with your treatment. If you are having vaginal dryness, you will want to discuss the above options with your oncologist.

Hair Loss

Certain chemotherapies cause hair loss, as discussed in chapter 9 on chemotherapy. For a majority of women, this is a devastating side ef-

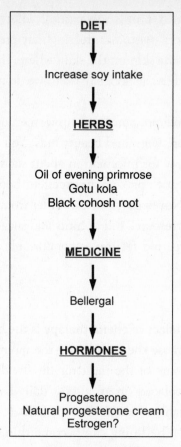

FIGURE 10.1

Sequential management of menopausal symptoms
in women with breast cancer

fect. As we discussed, chemotherapy does *not* cause permanent damage
to the hair follicle but rather a defect in the hair protein, which causes
it to break. The chemotherapy drugs given for breast cancer that usually cause the most significant hair loss are doxorubicin (Adriamycin),
paclitaxel (Taxol), Taxotere, and oral cyclophosphamide (Cytoxan).

If you are taking these drugs, you can have some loss of eyelashes,
eyebrows, and pubic hair, but this is rare even with chemotherapies
that cause scalp hair loss. In an attempt to reduce scalp hair loss in patients, some centers have used ice caps to freeze the scalp and prevent

blood flow to hair follicles. This is only partially effective and can cause you moderate discomfort. Also, the freezing may prevent the chemotherapy from reaching the skin on the skull where, theoretically, there could be cancer cells. For the above reasons, we do not use ice caps at our center.

Many centers do have programs to help women undergoing cancer treatment with makeup, wigs, and beauty aids. You may want to call your local cancer society for information about such offerings in your area. Or you might want to pick up an excellent book entitled *Beauty and Cancer* by Diane Noyes that you can order from your local bookstore. It is a wonderful resource full of hints and suggestions to get you through this difficult period feeling as comfortable and attractive as possible.

Mouth Problems

Another possible side effect of chemotherapy is the breakdown of oral tissue. This occurs because the cells lining the mouth, known as mucous membrane, are some of the most rapidly dividing tissues in the body. This lining is replaced on an almost daily basis, which makes these cells very vulnerable to chemotherapy (which, as you know, targets replicating cells). The lining can become thin, sensitive, and in extreme cases, the skin can ulcerate.

To guard against this side effect, it is important to practice good oral hygiene during your treatment, while taking special care not to irritate your gums. I recommend that you have a professional teeth cleaning before starting chemotherapy. I do not endorse having routine dental services done while you are receiving chemotherapy because of an increased risk of seeding the bloodstream with bacteria. I advise that you frequently brush your teeth and rinse your mouth with antiseptics, but discourage aggressive flossing. The sensitized mucous membranes are more susceptible to minor trauma and herpetic infection, the danger of which can be increased with flossing. With herpetic ulcers, we use local antiviral therapy. If your cancer treatment results in any of these side effects, you may be able to ease your discomfort by rinsing your mouth with a mixture of liquid benadryl and milk of magnesia.

Remember that your medical team wants to make your treatment as tolerable as possible. But the only way for them to know what your particular side effects are is for you to communicate them. Your nurse specialist is usually the best person to start with.

CHECKPOINTS

1. Who is my contact person to help me manage my side effects?
2. Should I get my dental work done before I start chemotherapy or radiation?
3. What local community resources are available for me regarding my hair loss?

11

Tamoxifen

Tamoxifen belongs to a class of medications known as selective estrogen receptor modulators (SERMs, for short). A number of cells in the human female contain receptors for estrogen or estrogen-like molecules: the breast, uterus, vagina, skin, brain, and ovaries. SERMs enter these cells through specific cell surface receptors and act like keys turning on or off certain cellular functions. For example, estrogen attaches to receptors on breast cells and stimulates them to take on cellular building blocks and divide. This is mediated through a network of intracellular proteins. Tamoxifen, on the other hand, enters the estrogen receptor site and turns this mechanism off. In the case of breast cancer cells that contain estrogen receptors, tamoxifen may actually send the cell into a programmed death cycle.

Tamoxifen is taken orally like other hormones. In spite of "turning off" breast cells, it acts like estrogen on other tissue and has positive effects on bone metabolism. And, like estrogen, it can lower cholesterol (see Table 11.1).

There have been long-term studies demonstrating that tamoxifen increases the cure rate of women with localized breast cancer, but controversy still continues to surround its use. Part of the controversy stems from a recent national clinical trial to determine whether ta-

	Tamoxifen	Estrogen	Explanation
Breast	−	+ + +	Estrogen stimulates breast epithelia proliferation.
Uterus	+ +	++++	Estrogen stimulates uterine lining slightly more than tamoxifen.
Skin	+	+ +	Estrogen increases tissue moisture.
Vagina	−	+ +	Estrogen stimulates vaginal proliferation and lubrication.
Bone	+ +	+ +	Both tamoxifen and estrogen help retain bone calcium.
Hot Flashes	−	+ +	Estrogen reduces hot flashes.

TABLE **11.1**

Benefits and liabilities of tamoxifen and estrogen

moxifen can prevent primary breast cancer in high-risk well women. As a result of this prevention trial, tamoxifen received heavy scrutiny and some negative press overstating its potential side effects for well women.

There is absolutely no question that tamoxifen is an extremely valuable treatment for women with breast cancer, and most women tolerate its modest side effects without major problems. At our centers, we have recently changed our recommendations regarding the length of time women should be taking tamoxifen following the local treatment of breast cancer. This is based on results of a major trial comparing five years versus ten years of taking tamoxifen following early breast cancer diagnosis. Five years of taking tamoxifen greatly reduced the systemic recurrence of breast cancer, but an additional five years added only expense and potential risk of uterine cancer with no change in potential cure.

Not all breast cancers respond to tamoxifen, however; the prediction of the response is based upon the presence of estrogen and progesterone receptors in the primary tumor. As noted above, women who take tamoxifen for five years after breast cancer diagnosis have a significantly higher cure rate than women who do not. However, continuing on tamoxifen for more than five years does not seem to add to the survival benefit or cure rate.

When tamoxifen trials were launched over ten years ago, we did not understand how tamoxifen really worked, and we still do not completely understand the process today. At the beginning, we thought that tamoxifen blocked estrogen production by the ovaries. The ovaries produce the majority of estrogen normally, while the adrenal glands and fatty tissue manufacture smaller amounts. Estrogen affects multiple organs, including the breast, uterus, skin, brain, liver, and vagina. Tamoxifen was believed to have antiestrogen effects as long as women were taking it. The effects were on both cancer cells and estrogen sensitive cells in various tissues. If women were to stop taking the tamoxifen, we thought the blockade would be removed and all the preventative good that it had done would be reversed. If this were the case, tamoxifen would be called a static agent. An analogy is a static antibiotic, which paralyzes bacteria, allowing white blood cells to come along and gobble them up. The counterpart is the cidal antibiotic, which kills bacteria on its own and does not need white blood cells to complete the job.

We thought that tamoxifen was a static cancer drug because it put cancer cells to rest. We have since learned that tamoxifen is a cidal agent. Tamoxifen actually gets incorporated into the cancer cell surface, becoming or stimulating an internal messenger inside the cancer cell that causes the cell in its next cycle to go into a cell death. We have learned that tamoxifen is not static at all but appears to directly disrupt the cancer cell's life cycle.

Since breast cancers are very heterogeneous, they are not all constructed in the same cellular way; about 60 percent of them contain hormone receptors, the others do not. Tamoxifen appears to be more helpful to women who have estrogen and progesterone hormone receptors in their tumors than to those who don't. However, within a given breast cancer, there may be cells that have more hormone receptors than others. Thus, tamoxifen may work only partially.

It is also possible that, over time, a population of cells that are hormone receptor positive may even evolve and become hormone receptor negative. In theory, this may be why women who receive a combination of chemotherapy and tamoxifen may have a better response than with either treatment alone. Usually, when chemotherapy and tamoxifen are given to a woman, they are given sequentially; chemotherapy, which kills off hormone receptor negative cancer cells, first, followed by tamoxifen that can then act on the hormone sensitive cancer cells that may be less susceptible to chemotherapy.

As stated, those women who have positive hormone receptors appear to be helped by tamoxifen more than those who have negative hormone receptors. The side effects of tamoxifen are very different from those of cytotoxic chemotherapy. Tamoxifen's side effects are primarily hormonal. For women close to menopause, tamoxifen often puts them into a full menopause, or a state of hormone withdrawal. Table 11.1 shows some of the expected effects of estrogen versus tamoxifen on estrogen receptive organs.

Women who seem to have the most difficulty with tamoxifen are those who are perimenopausal (about to begin menopause) and women on replacement estrogen who go off their dosages because of their recent breast cancer diagnoses. Most premenopausal women in their thirties and forties have almost no side effects with tamoxifen, and older women who are not on replacement hormones have little problem starting and taking tamoxifen.

The major potential toxic effect of tamoxifen is to the uterus. A small percentage of women have endometrial thickening, a stimulation to the glandular lining of the uterus, which, if left unchecked, can become cancerous. The chance of uterine malignancy as a result of taking tamoxifen is small, only about 1 percent, but your uterus should be monitored carefully with either an ultrasound or endometrial biopsy at the time of your annual pelvic exam if you are taking this drug.

Some of the irritating problems of tamoxifen can be vaginal dryness, hot flashes, and mild weight gain. These symptoms can be managed using a variety of remedies including natural products and/or herbs.

Women ask me, "Is this worth the risk of taking tamoxifen?" My answer is—*absolutely!* The potential survival benefit for those on tamoxifen is an average of 10 to 25 percent greater than it is for those women who do not take it; the uterine cancer risk is 1 percent, which can be monitored for and treated.

Tamoxifen was the first SERM developed, and we have over twenty years of experience using the drug. Recently, several other SERMs have been released, and more are presently being developed. The goal is to develop the "perfect" SERM that prevents breast cancer (or treats it) without stimulating the uterus, is good for the bones, and is good for lipid metabolism without causing hot flashes and other menopausal symptoms. This "perfect" SERM should be an excellent hormone replacement therapy for women entering menopause.

The newly released SERM, raloxifene hydrochloride (Evista), has been approved for the prevention of osteoporosis. It appears to not stimulate the breast and uterus, but we do not have sufficient data on its effect on breast cancer.

CHECKPOINTS

1. Is tamoxifen a potential therapy in my case?
2. What are the risks and benefits for me of taking tamoxifen?
3. Do I need to have my endometrial lining monitored while on tamoxifen? How and by whom?
4. If necessary, can my doctor refer me to a resource to help pay for the tamoxifen?

12

Clinical Research Trials

Progress in the treatment of breast cancer has been painfully slow. Treatment changes can only occur after physicians and their patients have been convinced that a new treatment is equal or superior to another already in use. This process of demonstrating whether a new therapy is better than the previous standard requires that women volunteer to participate in the testing of new medications and procedures. Such tests are known as clinical research trials.

These trials need to be done in an unbiased, fair way if their results are to be reliable. This requires that women be randomly entered into one of two or more treatment groups. Eventually, the outcomes of the women in different groups of the trial are compared against each other. Randomized clinical trials are responsible for the many recent advances in cancer treatment. Data drawn from clinical trials have shown that less surgery and radiation are as effective as more invasive mastectomies, that giving chemotherapy to women with local breast cancer prevents the appearance of metastatic disease, and that tamoxifen increases the cure rate in women with hormone positive breast cancer. The randomized clinical trial has eliminated physician and investigator bias, a major problem in trials comparing a new therapy with standard therapies.

The major breast cancer research group in this country and possibly the world is the National Surgical Adjuvant Breast and Bowel Project, known as the NSABP. This group, which involves surgeons and radiation and medical oncologists from all over North America, has conducted more than thirty randomized trials in breast cancer over the past thirty years. It has been the group most responsible for the progress that has been made in breast cancer treatment for North American women.

The women who have been willing to participate in these studies have made a significant contribution to medical progress for all of womankind while receiving the best therapy available. Each trial tested a new hypothesis, or possible truth, and the results then became a knowledge base for the next clinical trial. In order to show significant differences in therapy, several thousand women are needed to volunteer for each trial. These volunteers realize that they may be getting established or experimental treatment and will not be told which. They bravely participate with this degree of uncertainty. The pioneer women were those who agreed to go on trials comparing mastectomy to WLE or chemotherapy versus a placebo. These women didn't know if one treatment was more or less effective than the other, but agreed to help answer the question of which was the optimal therapy. Today, the trials compare what is the standard of practice, or "state of the art," to what *potentially* might be better. The difference in each treatment regime in trials today involves the sequencing of different therapies or the addition of a new drug.

There are many opportunities to participate in clinical research trials in which you would receive state of the art care. Those that are known for their cutting edge studies include the National Cancer Institute (NCI), which sponsors them through one of the major national groups such as National Surgical Adjuvant Breast Project (NSABP), Southwest Oncology Group (SWOG), or Cancer and Leukemia-Group B (CALGB). In order to participate, you must be willing to be randomized to a treatment group. You would be asked to sign very detailed informed consent forms that explain the research objectives and the risks and benefits involved.

There are also studies called pilot studies. These are done in a center that is running clinical research that is not NCI sponsored and is not randomized. They are often underwritten by pharmaceutical companies, entrepreneurial companies, or conducted at a university. There are safeguards in place in pilot studies to protect participating women as much as possible. These protocols are usually only for women with advanced disease who may be willing to place themselves at risk because of limited alternatives available to them at that late stage.

Human clinical trials are separated into three phases depending on the questions that each one is attempting to answer. *Phase I* testing is designed to determine if a promising treatment has acceptable tolerance in patients and at what dosage significant side effects appear. Once an agent, drug, or treatment has been proven safe, the *Phase II* testing quantifies the objective response rate; *objective* in this context means resulting in a measurable reduction in cancer. In women with breast cancer, both Phase I and Phase II testing is performed on those with metastatic disease. *Phase III* testing compares the standard treatment to a promising treatment that has gone through Phase I and Phase II testing. Most of the trials for women with newly diagnosed breast cancer are of the Phase III type.

My advice concerning clinical research is that you ask your doctors if you are eligible for any trials. Also inquire as to whether they participate as investigators in any studies or if there is a NSABP participating center near you. Your ability to participate may depend upon the type of health care delivery system you are in, so you will want to talk to your insurance company or HMO representative as well. In general, the next five to ten years should prove very exciting in the field of breast cancer clinical research because there are tremendous financial and scientific resources being devoted to the cause.

CHECKPOINTS

1. Am I eligible for a current nationally sponsored clinical research trial?
2. Do my doctors participate in clinical research? If yes, what type?
3. What NSABP protocol am I eligible for?
4. Is the therapy my doctors are recommending for me similar to any research arms of a clinical trial or pilot study?

13

Diet, Exercise, Herbs, and Vitamins

In this chapter, we will discuss diet, nutrition, and herbal dietary supplements and therapies that can reduce the side effects associated with cancer treatments and minimize your body's healing time. At our breast center, we have been fortunate to have an expert in Eastern medicine who provides us with a great deal of alternative treatment wisdom. Many women appreciate this holistic approach.

If there was one major weakness in my medical school training, it would be in the area of nutrition. From talking with other physicians, I know I am not alone in feeling this way. Traditionally, we viewed diseases as attacking the body from the outside, like an infectious agent. Nutrition and diet were not emphasized as critical to the battle in our study of Western medicine. We now know nutrition and the general state of our health are critical in preventing, fighting, and recovering from all illness, including breast cancer.

The information about the effectiveness of dietary supplements and herbal treatments has been studied and developed differently from the information about chemotherapy regimes. As discussed earlier, researchers study groups of people closely to determine the effectiveness of a particular dose or sequence of chemotherapy regimes compared to the best treatment plan already known. This information is published for a specialized audience of oncology doctors, who use the data in the treatment of their patients. But herbal and dietary supplements are rarely studied this way. Instead, people trained in other modes of healing use treatments that have been passed on from their teachers and seem to be useful in treating their patients. The time has come, however, for more traditional scientific testing of these herbal and supplementary therapies, and some preliminary work like this has begun.

Many of the women I see at the initial consultation following a diagnosis of breast cancer are partially convinced that they have caused their breast cancer either by poor diet, lack of exercise, excessive stress, and/or many of the other highly publicized but undocumented causes. There is no evidence that any particular agent or factor is responsible for breast cancer. Quite popular now are articles and even books suggesting breast cancer can be prevented, and even cured, by dietary and lifestyle changes. This approach has a certain appeal to us because it is simple and empowering, but unfortunately there is no evidence to support the claims.

Nor is there evidence that breast cancer results from a depressed immune system. Unfortunately, it appears that the human immune system cannot differentiate a breast cancer cell from a normal breast glandular cell even though it may have significant differences due to DNA derangement. For example, the development of the drug trastuzumab (Herceptin) is based on the overexpression (production) of a gene fragment that leads to increased amounts of a cell surface protein not found on normal breast cells. The host cannot recognize this abnormal cell and its increase in protein, but an antibody can be developed by using another species' immune system and then, through genetic engineering, that information can be transferred into a human antibody producing cell. These altered human cells then make an antibody against the cell surface protein. This antibody can destroy the cell and make it more susceptible to other agents.

The point is that breast cancer is not recognized by a normal immune system. As we develop more knowledge we may be able to manipulate the immune system through vaccines and genetically engineered proteins.

Your immune system is probably, almost certainly, just fine. If you require chemotherapy your immune system will be impaired temporarily, but this will be completely reversible and will not allow the cancer any advantage. Your immune system is important in preventing infection, and you need to take care of it and your body and its ability to heal through nutrition, vitamins, and exercise.

Diet

❧ We have been told for years that "we are what we eat." There is some truth to this, since our diet constitutes the building blocks for tissue repair and energy storage within our bodies. Accumulated evidence shows that certain dietary factors may contribute to problems associated with the rise in cardiovascular disease and a few cancers such as colon, liver, and possibly breast cancer. There is also growing evidence that certain environmental pollutants contribute specifically to estrogenic activity and thereby may contribute in some way to the rise of breast cancer. With this in mind, I recommend to our patients that they consider the following dietary suggestions:

Reduce Fat Intake to 20 Percent or Less of Your Daily Caloric Intake

Many studies have implicated an increase in total fat intake in the higher incidence of breast cancer. Of the twenty-five studies published since 1985 that examined diet and risk of breast cancer, ten studies found a statistically significant relationship between a high level of total dietary fat intake and the risk of breast cancer. One international study done in 1991 found that the United States had one of the highest intakes of fat grams per person per day (about 140 grams), and also had one of the highest rates of death from breast cancer.

These studies are retrospective and involve dietary questionnaires of women with breast cancer comparing them to women who have similar characteristics (case controls) without breast cancer. Some of these studies are population based, looking at average fat consumption of women in different populations versus their breast cancer incidence. These types of studies give indirect evidence at best. Prospective randomized dietary studies are extremely difficult and expensive to conduct. There are several in progress that may help us answer the question of dietary fat intake and breast cancer risk.

As we await these prospective studies to progress, the retrospective comparative studies do suggest a relationship between fat consumption and breast cancer.

Interestingly, in Italy, the consumption of olive oil, high in mono-unsaturated fatty acid, is much higher than in the United States, but the death rate from breast cancer is one-half of that in this country. One of the reasons for this may be that polyunsaturated fats, not mono-unsaturated fats, are consumed in high quantities in the United States but not in Italy.

An example of a population-based study is the observation found that when women emigrate from a country with a low incidence of breast cancer and low-fat intake to a country with a high incidence of the disease and high-fat intake, their breast cancer risk gradually rises and approaches the risk of that disease in the new country. An assumption is made that the causative variable in breast cancer is fat; however, this may not be the case. It may be something entirely unrelated, such as soy consumption or the lack of it. This is the problem with a retrospective population-based study.

Partially hydrogenated fats, used primarily to improve the shelf life of products, are the most harmful form of fat. Polyunsaturated fats, the kind that are always promoted as heart healthy, are next in line. In several animal studies, results showed that polyunsaturated fats such as those found in liquid vegetable oils—corn or safflower oils—can promote tumor growth.

Current theories suggest that an ideal diet might provide you with 10 percent of your calories from monounsaturated fats (in the form of canola or olive oil) and maybe 5 percent from supplemental oils. Mono-unsaturated fats seem to play a beneficial role in the management of blood cholesterol and, therefore, heart disease. It is important that you get *some* fats in your diet since they supply essential fatty acids for general health and tissue repair. Some of the foods that are a rich source of essential fatty acids are: wheat germ; fish, such as trout, salmon, and mackerel; seeds, such as flax, soy, and pumpkin; and nuts, such as walnuts and almonds. Olive oil and canola oil should be the only oils you use. Olive oil is unstable at high temperatures; therefore use canola oil for high temperature cooking and frying, and use olive oil for salads and light cooking only.

You can adopt the healthy, practical approach toward reducing your unhealthy fat intake by:

1. Using only monounsaturated fats in the form of canola or olive oil
2. Eliminating red meat from your diet as much as possible because animal fat accompanies muscle protein
3. Adding fish, such as salmon, trout, and mackerel, to your diet because it contains essential fatty acids that are necessary for your total health
4. Eating sweets such as cakes, cookies, and other dessert-type foods on rare occasions only

It is important to remember that some fat is essential in one's diet. Fat is also the most concentrated form of calories, yielding over twice as many calories per unit of weight as compared with carbohydrates and protein.

Increase the Percentage of Complex Carbohydrates in Your Diet

Complex carbohydrates include whole grains, vegetables, and fruits, which are high in dietary fiber. Researchers suggest there may be an association between increased dietary fiber and decreased breast cancer.

It has been hypothesized that the reason behind this correlation is that the fiber binds to excess estrogen in the intestinal tract and is then excreted. Diets high in fat can promote the growth of intestinal bacteria that allows the estrogen to be reabsorbed into the body. Thus, a high-fat/low-fiber diet decreases the excretion of estrogen, and women on this type of diet appear to be at an increased risk for breast cancer.

A good anticancer diet should include beans, grains, nuts, seeds, and brown, unpolished rice. Millet cereal is also a good source of protein and fiber. You can vary your diet by eating grains such as wheat, oat, and bran. Eat plenty of cruciferous vegetables such as broccoli, brussels sprouts, cabbage, radishes, cauliflower, kale, and collard greens.

A compound called indole-3-carbinol (I3C), which is a plant chemical obtained from cruciferous vegetables, changes the way estrogen is metabolized by converting estrogen into a metabolite other than the active form linked to cancer. Researchers believe that the reduced endogenous estrogen availability for breast ductal cells reduces the stimulation and production of genetic abnormalities leading to cancerous change. This phytochemical has also been shown to reduce the incidence of mammary cancer in mice. Another phytochemical, found in broccoli, has been found to increase the synthesis of specific enzymes that detoxify cancer-causing substances within the body.

Yellow, deep orange/red, and dark green vegetables and fruits, such as cantaloupe, carrots, pumpkin, squash, yams, peppers, kale, and lettuce, are high in vitamin A and beta-carotene, which may also protect the body against breast cancer by defending against oxidative damage. You'll want to include these in your diet as well.

Eat as Many Organically Grown Meats, Vegetables, Fruits, and Grains as Possible

Evidence is emerging from several studies that strongly suggests DDT-like pesticides and other organochlorines act like or cause the body to produce a carcinoma-promoting type of estrogen (xenoestrogen). This has raised a great deal of controversial attention as to the role that these xenoestrogens may play in regard to the rise in breast cancer.

One of the more provocative studies along this line was done by Dr. Elihu Richter of Hebrew University in Israel. When that country outlawed the use of certain DDT-like pesticides for several years, Dr. Richter found that the rate of breast cancer was reduced by 30 percent while around the world the rates had increased. The work by Dr. Devra Lee Davis at the Strang Research Laboratory in New York has strongly suggested that the DDT-like pesticides or organochlorines cause the body to produce a carcinoma-promoting type of estrogen (16 alpha hydroxyestone). Conversely, the "good" foods, micronutrients, and fats we have mentioned may actually reduce a woman's risk of developing breast cancer by reducing the more stimulatory estrogen metabolites.

Low intakes of fruits and vegetables have been linked epidemiologically to an increased risk of several cancers, including breast cancer. It has been found that people who consume more fruits and vegetables have less risk, and if cancer is diagnosed, these individuals have lower mortality rates. The overall benefits of consuming adequate amounts of fruits and vegetables on breast cancer are largely due to the antioxidants present, as well as the nonnutrient phytochemicals that appear to have protective qualities.

Eat Lots of Soy-Based Protein

It has long been known that Japanese and Chinese women eat much more soy than North Americans do, and that Japanese women, in particular, have significantly lower rates of breast cancer. In fact, in several international studies, Japan was found to have the lowest per capita rate of breast cancer of any country studied. A low-fat diet coupled with high intake of soy-based products may be one of the leading reasons for this. These results and other studies on soy have sparked the attention of the National Cancer Institute (NCI), which launched in 1990 a $3 million research program on soy and cancer. We are awaiting the results of this study.

How does soy possibly help to prevent cancer? The soy plant, like all plants, produces phytoalexins, chemicals used to defend the plant against disease, irradiation, drought, and other threats. These phytoalexins are not unique to the soybean plant, but one form, known as isoflavones, is found almost exclusively in soy. In the human bowel, isoflavones are converted by intestinal bacteria into phytoestrogens, or plant estrogens. One of these phytoestrogens, genistein, is about 1/100,000 as strong as the estrogen produced by the ovaries, but it does have the ability to lock onto estrogen receptors in the breast and elsewhere, blocking the activity of estradiol. Soy proteins then act as SERMs and compete with estradiol at various receptor sites in the female body.

This blocking action is the key factor in soy's effectiveness as a cancer preventative. During a woman's menstrual cycle, the ovary produces large amounts of estrogen, which affect cells all over the body. Estradiol, the ovarian estrogen, binds with estrogen receptors in the breast and stimulates new growth. For many women, this is one factor contributing to swollen and sometimes painful breasts prior to menstruation. This constant stimulation of breast tissue on a monthly basis for a period of thirty to forty years may lead to an increased risk of breast cancer. It is postulated that the soy phytoestrogens occupy breast estrogen receptor sites and prevent some of the stimulatory effect of ovarian estrogens. In this sense genistein and similar proteins may act like a "natural" form of tamoxifen or one of the other synthetic SERMs. Because of the population-based conclusions that soy perhaps can decrease breast cancer, there has been a major interest in increasing dietary soy intake among women.

One bit of caution in this regard. A group of scientists at the University of Illinois recently reported that genistein actually stimulated estrogen-dependent breast cancer cells in tissue culture when implanted into mice.* However, this appeared to be concentration dependent, with higher concentrations being inhibitory to breast cancer growth. Also, it is quite conceivable that the human female may convert genistein into a related SERM compound that is inhibitory.

Although the intake of soy has been associated with lower risk of incidence and mortality rates from breast cancer, not all studies are conclusive, and this area will require long-term evaluation in order for us to completely understand the diverse functionality of soy foods and their components.

Not only may genistein help reduce the risk of developing breast cancer, it also may have the ability to inhibit the growth of tumors that are being formed. In order to grow, tumors need a blood supply. The success of a tumor in gaining a foothold in the body depends on its ability to generate this blood supply through a process called angiogenesis. Genistein in soy acts as an antiangiogenesis agent and inhibits the formation of new blood vessels, thereby reducing a tumor's blood supply, eventually cutting off its nutrient source completely and causing it to die.

As if this were not significant enough, soy has other positive effects on the body. The isoflavones in soy can bring relief from hot flashes and night sweats thanks to their ability to help mute or stabilize the impact of your hormonal fluctuations during perimenopause and postmenopause. One source suggests that by adding 45 g (1.6 oz) of soy to your daily diet, you can reduce the frequency of hot flashes and night sweats by 40 percent without excessively stimulating breast tissue.

Soy products can be found in the form of soybeans, soy sprouts (similar to mung bean sprouts), soy nuts (sold as a snack food); and textured vegetable protein (TVP), which has a texture like ground beef

---

*Ching-Y Hsieh, R. C. Santell, et al., "Estrogenic Effects of Genistein on Growth of Estrogen Receptor Positive Human Breast Cancer (MCF-7 Cells) in Vitro and in Vivo," *Cancer Research* 58 (September 1, 1998): 3833–38.

when rehydrated from granular form. Tofu, soy flour, soy milk, soy protein powder, tempeh (a combination of soybeans and grains with a distinctive taste resembling mushrooms), and miso (a fermented soybean paste that is a great source for soup stock) are also good sources of soy. Soy sauce, a popular flavoring, is not a good source because it has a very high sodium content.

Let me say a few more words about protein in general. Proteins are essential for tissue repair, enzyme production, and cell reproduction. However, we have become protein gluttons, with the average North American consuming many times more protein than is necessary for daily living. The excess protein we ingest is simply broken down and stored as fat and glycogen, with the nitrogen molecule being eliminated through the kidney in the form of urea. Many of us can cut back on our protein intake with no adverse effects whatsoever.

But you should be sure as a cancer patient that you are providing your body with the protein it needs. If the body is stressed by cancer or its treatment, adequate protein is necessary for tissue repair and immune function. If this protein is not supplied by your daily diet, then healing will be retarded and the body will enter a catabolic state in which tissue breakdown may occur to supply essential amino acids. Therefore, soy would be an excellent protein source as well as nuts, beans, lentils, fish, and organic meat and eggs.

Foods You Should Avoid
In addition to reducing fat and nonorganically grown foods in your diet, you should avoid the following, whether or not you've had breast cancer.

Junk Foods, Processed Refined Food, Salt, Sugar, and White Flour
The refining process of sugar cane strips it of all its vitamins, minerals, and enzymes that the body needs to efficiently metabolize the sugar. Foods with refined sugars should be avoided for the following reasons:

1. Ingesting it will lower the immune system for several hours afterward.

2. Calcium will be given up by the bones in order to alkalize the sugar's acidity in the bloodstream (to buffer the unhealthy acidic state in the body created by the load of sugar in the system).

3. Sugar can cause a hormonal imbalance in the body.

You can substitute a small amount of blackstrap molasses, pure maple syrup, or fruit sweetener as natural sweeteners in place of sugar. Use whole wheat, rye, and other flours instead of white flour.

All Foods Containing Caffeine
Coffee, tea (except for herbal teas), colas, and chocolate all contain caffeine. Besides having a negative effect on breast tenderness and fibrocystic change, caffeine can, according to some studies, increase such menopausal symptoms as hot flashes.

Alcohol
Alcohol can affect liver function and have a dehydrating effect on the body. It can also have a depressing effect on the immune system. You should avoid it especially during chemotherapy. Although recent studies have shown an association between increased risk of breast cancer and alcohol consumption, the degree of risk and the mode of action are not yet understood.

Carbonated Drinks
Such drinks contain phosphorus, which causes the body to lose calcium. Women with breast cancer can have problems with calcium deficiency because of chemotherapy and premature menopause. Most of these drinks also contain high levels of sugar, which contribute to increases in insulin secretion and major fluctuations in blood sugar. You should cut back on these or avoid them altogether.

Supplements: Vitamins, Minerals, and Other Nutrients

❧ Vitamins function in the body as coenzymes and factors in cellular metabolism. In a perfect world, we would be able to obtain all the vitamins we needed from our foods. Since this isn't the case for most of us, we need to supplement our diets with *moderate* amounts of vitamins, minerals, and essential fatty acids.

A primary focus here is the additional support that your body will need during and after chemotherapy and/or radiation. More specifically, you will want to rid your body of the toxins and free-radical damage produced by both treatments. Your body must have a full spectrum of micronutrients in biologically available forms and appropriate proportions to assist your innate healing mechanisms as they work to correct disease conditions, to sustain your wellness, and to achieve optimum health.

Free radicals are unstable molecules that have the ability to attach to DNA and cause genetic damage. They are produced when the body

- performs normal aerobic exercise, especially vigorous exercise, as oxygen is utilized
- experiences an *oxidative burst* from white blood cells as they kill bacteria and viruses, and by which foreign proteins, or antigens, are neutralized. (Chronic inflammation, infections and other illnesses, and exposure to allergens contribute to the body's oxidant load.)
- detoxifies toxic substances, such as drugs, cigarette smoke, pollution, pesticides, and insecticides
- is exposed to chemotherapy and radiation

Oxidants are capable of stimulating cell division, a critical factor in mutagenesis and therefore carcinogenesis, or cancer growth. They can stimulate cell division of a mutated cell having a damaged DNA strand, perhaps as a result of free radical exposure. This causes cell replication, which allows for the passage of abnormal DNA to daughter cells, an important factor in carcinogenesis. It is believed that antioxidants exert their protective effect by decreasing oxidative damage to DNA and by decreasing abnormal increases in cell division.

Overall, free radicals have been implicated in the cause of at least fifty diseases (including cancer). Diet may account for as much as 35 percent of all human cancers. However, epidemiological evidence consistently relates low antioxidant intake or low blood levels of antioxidants with increased cancer risk. Therefore, I strongly suggest that you pay attention to the elimination of free radicals. It has been reported that low dietary intake of fruits and vegetables, which contain antioxidants and other essential vitamins and minerals, increases the risk of many types of cancers. So, in addition to the diet already mentioned, I recommend that all women who are undergoing some form of anticancer therapy take the following antioxidants: vitamin C plus bioflavonoids, beta-carotene, selenium (taken with vitamin E), and a coenzyme known as CoQ10.

Table 13.1 gives the antioxidants that are recommended for women who are going through chemotherapy and/or radiation. The supplements listed in Table 13.2 illustrate the recommended doses after conclusion of chemotherapy and/or radiation. Generally, the posttreatment protocol increases vitamin doses and adds calcium and magnesium.

There is an ongoing debate regarding the potential of antioxidants to protect cancer cells from the desired cytotoxic or killing effects of

Beta-carotene	10,000–25,000 units
Coenzyme Q10	100–200 mg
Selenium	100–200 mcg
Vitamin E	400–800 IU
Vitamin C plus bioflavonoids	1,000–2,000 mg

TABLE 13.1

Daily vitamin supplements during treatment

Beta-carotene	50,000 units
Selenium	200 mcg
Vitamin E	400–800 IU
Vitamin C plus bioflavonoids	2,000–4,000 mg
Multivitamins (without iron)	1 tablet
Calcium/magnesium	1,500 mg calcium/ 750 mg magnesium

TABLE 13.2

Daily vitamin supplements after treatment

chemotherapy and radiation. To my knowledge, there are no controlled studies to date that have tested this hypothesis. Until we have a definitve answer regarding the use of antioxidants with chemotherapy and radiation, we are recommending the following modifications:

1. During the five to seven weeks of radiation, discontinue antioxidants except on the weekends, using the lower dose recommended in Table 13.1.
2. During chemotherapy, discontinue antioxidants two days before chemotherapy treatment and wait to re-start them two days after each treatment. If the chemotherapy regimen requires oral cyclophosphamide for fourteen days, discontinue the antioxidants during the entire fourteen days, with an additional two days on the end of each cycle.

Vitamin C plus Bioflavonoids

Vitamin C is considered the most important water-soluble antioxidant in all fluids surrounding the cells in your body. More than a hundred studies have reported that reduction in cancer risk is associated with a diet high in vitamin C. Foods high in vitamin C are potatoes, peppers, peas, tomatoes, broccoli, brussels sprouts, cabbage, cauliflower, kale, and parsley, as well as most fruits and melons.

Bioflavonoids are crystalline compounds that give food their great taste and bright colors. They are essential for the absorption of vitamin C. In addition, flavonoids in food and herbs have been demonstrated to have anti-inflammatory, antiallergic, antiviral, antiaging, and anti-carcinogenic effects due to their antioxidant properties. The use of bioflavonoids may also inhibit estrogen synthesis. The richest food sources of bioflavonoids are the inner peel and pulp of citrus fruit; the skin of grapes, cherries, and berries; and green tea polyphenols, quercetin, and proanthocyanidins.

Beta-carotene

Beta-carotene is a powerful antioxidant providing protection to all lipid-rich tissues in the body, including the skin; the mucous membrane of the mouth, nose, throat, and lungs; the soft tissue and linings of the digestive tract, kidneys, and bladder; and breast tissue. It is converted into usable vitamin A mainly in the upper intestinal tract. Several studies have shown that an increase in dietary beta-carotene may significantly decrease the risk of breast cancer.

The ability of the body to utilize carotene varies with the food and the form in which the food is ingested. Cooking, pureeing, or mashing vegetables ruptures the cell membranes and therefore makes the carotene more available for absorption. Carotene is abundant in carrots, but it is present in even higher concentration in green leafy vegetables such as beet greens, spinach, and broccoli.

Selenium (Taken with Vitamin E)

Selenium is an essential mineral found in small amounts in the body. It is a natural antioxidant that works closely with vitamin E in some of its metabolic actions and in the promotion of normal body growth and fertility. Dr. Julian E. Spallholz of the Veterans Administration Hospital in Long Beach, California, has demonstrated through experiments with mice that selenium may increase resistance to disease by increasing the number of antibodies that neutralize toxins.

Good food sources of selenium are brewer's yeast, fish and shellfish, grains, and cereals. Organ and muscle meats and dairy products are also good sources, but they are not recommended for women on an anti-cancer diet. So, we suggest that women stick to the meatless and dairy-free sources.

Coenzyme Q10

CoQ10 is a nutrient normally produced by the body. It is a key factor in energy production in the mitochondria, known as the powerhouse, of every cell in the body. When CoQ10 is low, it is like having so little gas remaining in your gas tank that your car sputters and misfires. Natural production of CoQ10 drops as we age. It is also low in people with a serious illness, compounding the deficiency associated with aging. This appears to be especially true for persons with cancer. Fortunately, our supply of CoQ10 is easily restored by oral consumption.

Several medical reports on the use of CoQ10 in the treatment of breast cancer have been positive and interesting, but like much of the research in the nutritional field, they lack rigorous scientific analysis. In addition, CoQ10 replacement therapy has been used extensively in Japan for many years, especially for treating heart disease. It is increasingly being used by physicians in the United States. It is also widely available over-the-counter and appears to be nontoxic and without side effects.

Other Recommended Supplements

Multivitamin and Multimineral Supplements

You should start taking a multiple vitamin and mineral supplement at least one month after your treatments are completed. You must provide your body with a full spectrum of micronutrients in biologically available forms and appropriate proportions to assist your innate healing mechanisms in correcting disease conditions.

Multiple Enzyme Digestive Formula
You can take this with meals to help aid in digestion. This is especially helpful for women who are undergoing or have recently undergone any form of chemotherapy. The effects of the drugs used will often compromise the function of your digestive tract for some time and therefore will adversely affect your ability to digest foods and nutrients properly and completely. A multiple enzyme digestive formula will aid in your absorption of nutrients, important in maintaining health and proper functioning of the body.

Calcium and Magnesium (Taken Together in a 2:1 Ratio)
These minerals are important in helping you maintain and create bone mass. It is particularly important for you to take them after chemotherapy and radiation treatments.

For reasons that are not clear to me, women undergoing chemotherapy have a significant loss of bone during this period of time. Because it is difficult to digest, many women find it hard to take calcium during chemotherapy. However, if it is tolerable, taken during this time it may be beneficial. The chemotherapy drugs may affect the osteoblastic cells that are constantly replacing reabsorbed bone. This loss is small in relation to one's total bone mass, perhaps 1 to 2 percent, but it is difficult to replace later.

There are medications to help correct osteoporosis. One class of medications is called biphosphonates. A group of German doctors recently performed a randomized clinical trial using a biphosphonate in women with newly diagnosed breast cancer. The groups of women receiving the biphosphonate known as clondrinate had a significantly lower systemic recurrence rate compared with the women who did not receive the medication. Other breast cancer research groups are in the process of repeating the experiment to see if the results can be confirmed. If so, this would be a major breakthrough in that the biphosphonates have few side effects. The common biphosphonate used in North America at this time is alendronate, or Fosamax.

There are a number of forms of calcium that are available. Some are more absorbable than others, including calcium citrate, or microcrystalline hydroxyapatite concentrate (MCHC), which is a crystalline complex providing calcium, phosphorus, and organic factors naturally present in healthy bone. Some calcium preparations have a small amount of vitamin D added.

One of the richest food sources of calcium is seaweed. You can eat it daily as a salad, vegetable, condiment, or seasoning. Other rich sources are dark green, leafy vegetables such as kale, collards, beet greens, cabbage, brussels sprouts, and broccoli. Additional sources of calcium include tofu, molasses, and almonds. Most kinds of beans, fish (such as salmon with bones and halibut), berries, raisins, and some grains are also good sources you can include in your diet.

Essential Fatty Acids
These are critically important but are largely absent from American food sources, since they are damaged or destroyed during modern food processing. As a result, most Americans are chronically deficient, often seriously so, in the daily consumption of EFAs.

EFAs are of vital importance since they maintain the fluidity and flexibility of cells and regulate the passage of substances into and out of cells. They also act as building blocks for important hormonelike compounds called prostaglandins, which are involved in regulating blood pressure, cardiovascular function, fat metabolism, inflammatory response, and immune and nervous system function.

When taken as a supplement over a period of six months or more, the essential fatty acids gradually drive out or replace much of the damaged and hydrogenated fat that has been used by all living cells of the body in the absence of high-quality fats. I recommend that you take both flaxseed oil and evening primrose oil, alternating every two weeks to facilitate this process. Use one for two weeks and then switch to the other. Dosages should be up to 1,000 mg of evening primrose oil or one tablespoon of flaxseed oil per day.

Antitumor and anticancer agents called lignans are also found in flaxseed in a quantity that is between seventy-five and eighty times greater than any other food. Researchers have discovered that lignans reduce the sex hormone bioavailability in the same way as the soy isoflavones do. In other words, they can help block estrogen from breast tissue, thereby inhibiting growth of estrogen-sensitive tumors. In addition, lignans contain a substance (a precursor to butyric acid) that induces differentiation of cells, thereby inhibiting cancer cell proliferation. Lignans can lower LDL levels significantly and may prevent bone loss as well.

One tablespoon of flaxseed is roughly equivalent to one serving of soy. You can also grind the flaxseeds in a coffee grinder and sprinkle them on your cereal, or soak them overnight and drink the liquid and seeds for breakfast.

Until more research is done on the diet and cancer, it is impossible to say exactly how much soy and flaxseeds a woman should take following the conclusion of her conventional Western treatments. One estimate is that 200 mg of soy equals 0.3 mg of pharmaceutical estrogen. Another estimate is that half a cup of soybeans and two soybean snacks are equivalent to about 200 mg of plant estrogen. I know this may not be the firm answer you are looking for here, but it is all we have to go on until further tests are run.

Before leaving diet and nutrition, I would like to conclude with what I call "The Cheeseburger Talk." I believe moderation and some flexibility are important in regard to one's diet. An occasional digression is acceptable. Remember, your stomach and small bowel do not see that cheeseburger or delectable dessert the way your eyes and taste buds do. When the cheeseburger enters the small bowel for absorption, it is already broken down into small molecules of fat, protein, and carbohydrates. The body, especially the healing body, needs some fat, protein, and carbohydrates, as discussed earlier. I believe the purity of ingredients over time is very important and that hormones along with additives for color and preservation may be potentially harmful. But, an occasional giving in to a craving is acceptable, and one does not need to have a major guilt attack over it. The same is true for alcohol on rare occasions. The key is moderation.

Herbs

Herbal medicine is the most ancient form of health care known to humankind. Herbs have been used in all cultures throughout history to ensure good health and nurse people back from illness. Native American cultures carry an abundance of healing wisdom as do European traditions, from the Welsh to the Sicilian. There are a number of highly developed medical systems around the world that today utilize medicinal plants in their healing work. These include ancient systems such as ayurveda from India and traditional Chinese medicine.

Extensive scientific documentation now exists concerning the beneficial use of herbs for health conditions, including premenstrual syndrome, indigestion, insomnia, heart disease, cancer, and HIV. Modern medicine is well aware of their benefits, with approximately 25 percent of all prescription drugs still derived from trees, shrubs, or herbs. Some are made from plant extracts. Others are synthesized to mimic a natural plant compound. The World Health Organization notes that of 119 plant-derived pharmaceutical medicines, about 74 percent are used by modern medicine in ways that correlate directly with their traditional uses as plant medicines by native cultures.

Other herbs have recently been discovered to aid in the treatment of more modern ills. For example, Taxol, a chemotherapy agent, is derived from the Pacific yew tree. Penicillin is derived from a mold. Aspirin, although now made synthetically, was first derived from the bark of the willowgreen tree. Digitalis comes from foxglove. Curare, an extract from a South American tree, was used by natives to paralyze animals during hunting. Today, modern anesthesiologists use this herb as a muscle relaxant during surgery.

At our center, I recommend herbs to women for several reasons: to boost their immune systems, to help minimize the side effects of chemotherapy and radiation, to increase their general energy and sense of well-being, and to manage any menopausal symptoms they might have. This recommendation is supported by a recent article in *The Journal of the American Medical Association (JAMA)* that reported the use of Chinese herbs as an important component of anticancer protocols. Life expectancy increased for patients with rapidly advancing cancers when Chinese herbs were added to their treatment plan, and their life quality also improved.

As helpful as herbs are, you need to be careful in how you take them. We are fortunate at our centers to have a licensed herbalist who works with our patients. There are a number of recent books written by knowledgeable herbalists that can help. Many health food stores and pharmacies have contacts who are knowledgeable in this ancient but revived area of medicine. As I stated earlier in regard to the similar situation with soy, some of the herbal remedies for menopausal symptoms have phytoestrogen activity. It would appear that they are safe in small amounts, but one must be careful not to overdose.

I have seen excellent results in those women who have chosen to use herbal remedies as an adjunct to modern medical treatments. They seem to experience fewer side effects, have more energy, and recover faster between each chemotherapy treatment than those women who do not use herbs and supplements. After women using herbs have completed Western medical treatments, including surgery, their recovery time also appears to be shortened.

If you are interested in looking into herbal medicines, seek a professional, an herbalist who has been extensively trained and licensed to be your guide and help you choose the right herbal therapy to address your specific needs.

Exercise

✌ The benefits of aerobic exercise to total health have been known for years. These benefits include weight control, cardiovascular fitness, and lowering of blood pressure. Aerobic exercise reduces stress and is generally energizing as well. My own observations lead me to conclude that chemotherapy slows your body's metabolism, which can result in mild weight gain and a generalized feeling of chronic fatigue. If you have a regular schedule of aerobic exercise, it will speed your body's recovery from chemotherapy and more rapidly return your metabolism to its normal state. But you need to be flexible and listen to your body during this time. Your body will let you know when the energy you have is needed for recovery as opposed to exercising. It is not something to feel guilty about if you find you cannot keep up with a regular exercise routine during treatment.

What do I mean by aerobic exercise? This is the "slow burn" type of exercise that requires at least thirty minutes, three to five times per week to have a visible beneficial effect. It should increase your heart rate during the exercise to approximately 70 percent of your predicted maximum heart rate. Your maximum predicted heart rate is usually calculated by subtracting your age from 220. For example, if you are fifty years old, the heart rate that you want to achieve during your exercise sessions would be calculated as follows: 220 minus 50 equals 170; 70 percent of 170 equals 119.

What type of exercise you choose to do depends on your lifestyle, weather conditions, and any physical limitations you might have, particularly related to your ongoing therapy. Fast walking, jogging, and swimming are the standard options, but thanks to mechanical technology we now have numerous exercise machines that are easy on the joints and allow you to do a secondary activity simultaneously, if you like, such as watching television or reading.

Epidemiological evidence suggests that cumulative exposure to ovarian hormones increases the risk of breast cancer. It is also known that aerobic exercise can modify menstrual cycle patterns and alter ovarian hormone production. Leslie Bernstein and her coworkers at the University of Southern California have demonstrated that four hours per week of physical exercise reduces a woman's risk of breast cancer by as much as 50 percent.* Clearly, this study suggests that young women can modify their breast cancer risk with physical exercise as part of their healthy lifestyle.

CHECKPOINTS

1. What is my physician's philosophy with regard to taking supplemental vitamins and herbs?
2. Is nutritional and dietary counseling appropriate and available for me?
3. What action should I take if I am not at my ideal weight?

---

*Leslie Bernstein et al., "Physical Exercise and Reduced Risk of Breast Cancer in Young Women," *Journal of the National Cancer Institute* 86, no. 18 (1994): 1403.

14

The Mind and Body Connection

All too often in the past, the traditional Western medical model didn't consider that an illness involves the *total* human being. But now there is evidence that the mind and the body are interconnected through a myriad of protein messengers that are continually acted on by hormones and neurotransmitters. We have also seen how the balance between the mind and body can affect the way our immune system responds to insult, injury, or disease. To separate or compartmentalize an illness from the rest of you and treat one part of the body as if it represents the totality of you, we now know, is a major mistake.

This chapter is not written to justify a holistic approach to your healing but simply to state fact. A holistic approach is necessary. Breast cancer is a very complex disease that involves genetics, hormones, nutrition, immunology, personality, lifestyle, and sexuality. To address only the physical cancer without exploring the rest of this picture is shortsighted. My experience is that women are more likely to seek out complementary healing approaches on their own if their doctors address only the *involved organ* and not the entire person. Complementary healing approaches may be helpful, but they have a much more positive effect if they are incorporated as part of a comprehensive plan.

One of the most promising areas of research in complementary healing approaches is the integration of support, which can be from your comprehensive medical team, a loving family, your psychological group, or a competent psychotherapist. A recent study conducted by Stanford University showed that women with breast cancer who attended ongoing support groups had better outcomes than a matched group of women who were not involved in a support group.* This type of research is difficult to do because there are so many variables to understand and control. Much of the outcome information involved issues that measured the participant's quality of life rather than the specific extent of her disease.

My own observations indicate that patients who utilize a support network, including their therapeutic team, a support group, and often some individual psychotherapy, seem to do better. All of these different sources of support help them cope better with anxiety and fear, reducing any depression they may experience. When women take the opportunity to put their lives into better balance during their cancer ordeal, they often reap unexpected benefits.

It may be difficult for you *not* to take a holistic approach to your illness. This is because, usually, when a woman develops breast cancer, her priorities change. She may see that a negative, unfulfilling relationship may not be worth working at anymore, or a material goal may not seem as fulfilling. Breast cancer can cause a woman to change her job, write a book, take up an old passion she had never focused on, develop new friendships, open up locked closets, and make new starts. Breast cancer is not a chosen passage but is the kind of path that can transform a person in a very positive way. Be open and welcoming to the new desires, hopes, and dreams you may encounter along the way.

---

*D. Speigel et al., "Effect of Psychological Treatment on Survival of Patients with Metastatic Breast Cancer," *Lancet 2* (1989): 888.

Their insight and experience make women who have navigated the journey through cancer excellent guides for newly diagnosed women. You can connect with others who have experienced what you are going through on an informal basis, but support groups, hospitals, and community programs also offer many opportunities for you to meet and share your experiences. Reaching out for assistance at a time when you are in crisis often requires energy and persistence. But I strongly suggest that you overcome any resistance you might have and reach out. The benefits are many.

All in all, the best reaction to stress is change and resolution, even though most of us want to just hold on to our life and habits as we know them until the stress is resolved. Life is stressful in and of itself. Having breast cancer adds a painful and frightening new dimension. What is often detrimental to one's health is remaining in a *chronic* unresolved state of mind that can become emotionally, psychologically, and physically depleting. This continuous depletion can weaken the body's capacity to fight disease.

With the current push for retaking control of one's life and disease, it is common for cancer patients to wonder how things went wrong. As a result of this line of thought, some women feel they may be responsible for their cancer. *I do not agree.* Can one's choices cause breast cancer? I do not believe so. Most of us can look back three to five years and identify a stressful period in our life: the death of a parent, marital problems, or difficulty with teenagers. Today, there is no evidence that these life events cause or have a major contribution to the development of cancer.

However, I do believe that attitude is an important factor in every patient's outcome. I believe there is something to the healing properties of a "strong will to live." There is emerging research on spiritual and emotional aspects of recovery and healing that will give us more insight into this mystery of the human spirit. I think it is valuable for women to feel they have as much control as possible over their recovery and health.

On the other hand, it is natural for women with newly diagnosed breast cancer to feel frightened, anxious, and depressed. How can you help but feel some of these emotions in the face of a life-threatening illness? Nevertheless, support groups can be very helpful to you while you are working through such feelings. Women in similar situations can share their experiences openly and can offer you new ways to cope and to try to change perceived threats into challenges. Not only do many of my patients find these support groups helpful in terms of fighting cancer, but many of them forge lasting friendships with others in them.

To find a support group in your area, contact the hospital or medical system you are involved with, the American Cancer Society, Y-Me, the Wellness Community, and other organizations. The "Resources" section at the back of this manual will help you get started.

Some women prefer individual psychotherapy during this crisis or along with their group experience. Often, the diagnosis of breast cancer coincides with life's other challenges or is the cause of them. Individual psychotherapy can provide you with many options regarding how to adjust, cope, and change in the face of them.

Priorities of many women change dramatically during the crisis of breast cancer. I have seen many patients take a look at their values and self-image in a way they really never have before. They struggle with issues of their own desirability, particularly where sexual feelings are concerned. We have had the privilege, at our center, to work with Wendy Schain, E.Ed., a renowned expert on psychosocial and sexual issues for women with breast cancer. As Wendy often states, "How can you *not* address sexual issues when discussing breast cancer? A woman's breast is a sex organ in our society!"

With the immediate crisis of breast cancer, you may find that your sexual desire and libido have markedly decreased. Many breast cancer patients suddenly have intense mixed feelings about what their breasts have meant to them as sources of pleasure for themselves and their lovers. You could very well have to cover this psychological and emotional territory along with physical changes from surgery and radiation and possible hormonal changes from chemotherapy and tamoxifen.

To say the least, if you are in a long-term relationship, this can be a difficult period for you and your partner. Open support and communication, as well as understanding and patience, are critical for you during this time. Your partner may need support of his/her own as well. Dealing with your mood changes, depression, and physical needs can be trying over a long period of time, and while your partner may want to help, he/she often doesn't know what to do. He/she may have his/her own anxiety, fear, and anger to work through.

I encourage spouses and significant others to be involved in the whole educational and therapeutic process, since it is usually very helpful, with the approval of you, the patient. However, in some cases, women choose to go through their experience without the support of others, a solo journey. I have observed many women successfully navigate the journey alone. You must do what feels right for you.

CHECKPOINTS

1. What support groups are in my area? Is the group for women with breast cancer only, or is it open to all cancers? Does the group focus on newly diagnosed patients, or is it open to people who have had recurrences? What is the average age of the participants? Is a support group available for significant others?
2. Should I consider individual psychotherapy regarding coping and related life issues affected by the cancer and the treatment? Can my physician recommend a psychotherapist who has experience with patients with cancer and/or loss issues?
3. What does my physician think is the correlation between the mind and the body and healing?

15

Genetic Risk

All cancer is genetic. That is to say, that in order for a normal cell to convert to a cancerous cell, a genetic mishap must occur. These genetic mishaps, or mutations, occur quite frequently and are usually of little consequence unless the event occurs at a critical location on one of the chromosomes. A single mutation does not lead to a cancer. Cancer results from two to three separate events over time. For many women breast cancer can be the result of several random chance occurrences, or genetic mishaps—in short, just bad luck. This may explain the presence of certain precancerous conditions such as atypical lobular neoplasia found in biopsies. These conditions may represent the cells' first or second mutation. Once cells are "primed," it only takes the final mutation to develop into cancer.

On the other hand, some women are predisposed to breast cancer because they have inherited one or several gene mutations. In this case, the "deck is stacked," so to speak, and only a single final genetic mishap is needed to convert a susceptible cell into cancer. In these predisposed women, the odds of developing breast cancer are greatly increased.

But soon we hope to even the odds in fighting the disease in these more predisposed women. Our knowledge of human genetics is increasing every day. Internationally, researchers are attempting to unravel the twenty-three chromosome pairs in each cell, along with their genetic codes. What has been expected to take decades to accomplish in genetic research is rapidly progressing ahead of schedule at this time. The hope is that, with the unraveling and understanding of the human genome, gene therapy will soon be available as a preventative strategy for those women who have a predisposing genetic abnormality.

Since a large number of human diseases have a genetic basis, we are certain to see major medical breakthroughs in the near future. Breast cancer should be among the diseases benefited by this research in genetics, and let's hope there will be a *cure*.

About 90 percent of breast cancer appears to be the sporadic type, which means the cancer occurs randomly without an underlying inherent defect in the patient's cells. However, 10 percent of women with breast cancer fall into the hereditary type who receive a defective gene from one of their parents that leads to a breast cancer later in life. Looking to narrow down the site at which cancer begins, scientists have studied over 1,000 separate families and their chromosomes, identifying several genetic defects. At present, these studies are expensive and laborious, but they should lead to the development of simpler testing and, ultimately, to the genetic source of cancer.

The first genetic abnormality that has been discovered to cause increased susceptibility to breast cancer has been labeled BRCA-1. It resides on the seventeenth chromosome and is an autosomal dominant defect. The defect is on one of the twenty-two non-sex-determining chromosome pairs, called autosomes, and, because it is dominant, requires only one of the two paired seventeenth chromosomes to be affected to manifest the cancer susceptibility. When a disorder requires both of the chromosomes in a pair to have the defect, it is known as recessive.

Researchers have hundreds of separately identified and thoroughly studied families with this BRCA-1, autosomal dominant defect. Approximately 60 to 90 percent of women with this defect will go on to have a final converting event and develop breast cancer. Moreover, breast epithelial cells are not the only susceptible cells. Between 25 and 60 percent of women with BRCA-1 will develop ovarian cancer. Since this is an autosomal defect, the children of an affected person have a 50 percent chance of inheriting the defective gene because when a person makes germ cells, eggs or sperm, only one of each pair of seventeenth chromosomes goes into each germ cell. This reduction of chromosomes is called meiosis. Males and females inherit the defect. Males with the defect do not develop breast cancer but do have a significantly higher incidence of prostate cancer.

Scientists have also discovered the next defective gene to contribute to an increase in breast cancer susceptibility, which they naturally called BRCA-2. The incidence of BRCA-2 appears to be slightly less than BRCA-1. BRCA-2 is autosomal dominant also and resides on the thirteenth chromosome. Initially, it was believed that the presence of the BRCA-2 gene defect did not appear to increase risk for ovarian cancer. However, it is now clear that these mutations do, in fact, increase the risk of ovarian cancer, perhaps by as much as 20 to 25 percent. This is not as high as with the mutations in BRCA-1, but significant nonetheless. It also appears that men with the defect have an increased incidence of breast cancer. The differences between BRCA-1 and BRCA-2 are listed in Table 15.1.

Our understanding of the genetics of cancer will most likely increase tremendously in the next few years. Current research will be outdated

	Percent of Breast Cancers	Chromosome	Type	Female Cancers	Male Cancers
BRCA-1	≈5%	17	Autosomal Dominant	Breast 60–90% Ovary 25–60%	Prostate
BRCA-2	≈3%	13	Autosomal Dominant	Breast 60–90% Ovary 25%	Breast

TABLE 15.1

Breast cancer gene defects

in only months because of how much and how rapidly data are now accumulating.

Here are some general principles that may help you understand cancer at the cellular level and that won't change over time. Genes are responsible for the production of proteins. Cancer is caused by the production of proteins that, in excess, stimulate uncontrolled cellular replication or the abnormal function of specific proteins that guard against cells going out of control. Gene defects that produce either type of protein in abnormal quantities or with deficits in function can lead to cancer.

There are three types of gene defects that appear to lead to cancer:

1. *Oncogene production.* This type of mutation leads to the production of proteins giving rise to the malignant transformation of the cell. An example is the Her-2/neu oncogene.
2. *Tumor suppressor gene defect.* This type of gene functions normally to produce proteins that protect cells against malignant transformation. When the gene gives rise to defective or absent proteins, cancers occur. This defect occurs only when both chromosomes are affected. An example is the P53 gene. The P53 gene is interesting because when a cell's genetic material is threatened, for example, by a virus or radiation, the P53 gene is activated and makes a protein that prevents the cell from dividing. Any defects in the genes resulting from the "attack" are repaired. Only then can the cell divide again; otherwise, it goes on to die without passing on the faulty genes. When no proteins are produced, however, a mutation can occur and run its course through to the development of cancer.
3. *Mutator genes.* These abnormal genes accelerate the production of oncogenes or defective tumor suppressor genes.

While we wait for more breakthroughs, doctors obtain information continuously from individual women's cancers and blood. Commercial genetic testing for breast cancer genes is now available as well. There are some ethical, legal, social, and medical issues created by this newly available genetic information that we all should address. Once armed with this patient information, the medical community must be prepared to counsel women on strategies of surveillance, prevention, and interventions. To give women critical information about increased breast cancer risks without action plans would only be an anxiety-provoking injustice. This new information availability raises concerns about confidentiality involving employers, the insurance industry, and the government.

At a recent national meeting for breast cancer researchers, a true story was told of a young woman who was a member of a possible BRCA-1 family that had been studied by researchers. Since this was a research study, it was not clear if and when she would receive results of the testing, so she had decided to have prophylactic bilateral mastectomies based on her family history alone. While getting preoperative blood work at the hospital, she stopped by the research lab. She explained to the research assistant about her upcoming surgery. The assistant promptly looked up her family file and told the woman that she was BRCA-1 negative. You can imagine her response—first relief, then elation, then guilt for not having what others in her family had. Finally, she was angry; angry at not being informed of her BRCA-1 negativity.

Women with newly diagnosed breast cancer are concerned about any possible risk to their daughters and sisters. If a woman does not appear to be in a family that has breast cancer in approximately half the women on one side, then she probably does not have either the BRCA-1 or BRCA-2 gene.

It is helpful to create a family chart for your physicians and for your own records to determine if such a pattern exists. You will be called the index case, and you will start with your two parents and two sets of grandparents. Then you can fill in any aunts, uncles, and siblings, listing any diseases, cancers, and causes of death for any of the deceased. Figure 15.1 is an example that will be helpful when you record your own family history. Your own family will have its own configuration, of

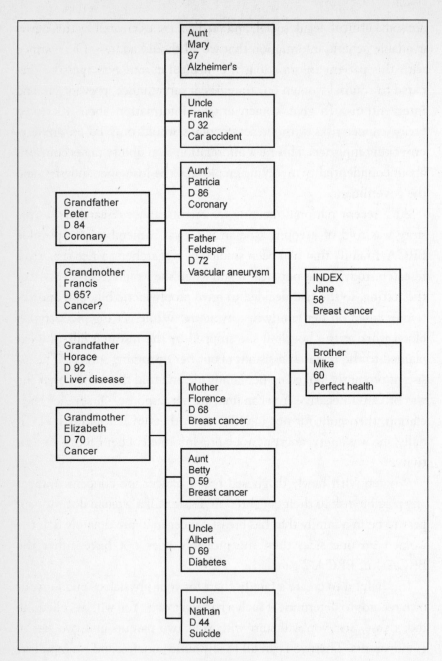

FIGURE 15.1

A sample family tree for cancer risk

course. For your record keeping, include the initials of relatives and their ages, the date of death and cause, and diseases.

Many women are understandably concerned about the risk of a second breast cancer. If your cancer is ductal in type and you do not have hereditary breast cancer in your family and you have no associated lobular neoplasia, your risk for recurrence is close to the average woman's risk (greater than a 12 percent lifetime risk or 0.5 percent per year). However, if you have lobular breast cancer or associated lobular neoplasia (LCIS or atypical lobular hyperplasia), your risk of developing a second breast cancer is higher. This is approximately 1.5 percent to 2 percent per year or a 30 percent lifetime risk. Mutations in BRCA-1 have been associated with a 25 to 30 percent risk of a second breast cancer within five years of the first diagnosis, and it is assumed that mutations in BRCA-2 are associated with comparable risks. In addition, mutations in either BRCA-1 or BRCA-2 make it ten times more likely that a woman with breast cancer will later on develop cancer of the ovary. Table 15.2 summarizes your risk. From this figure, you can determine what decisions you may need to make regarding further preventative measures to avoid a breast cancer recurrence.

Presently, there is only one laboratory offering full analysis of BRCA-1 and BRCA-2 outside of specific research projects. The test performed by this laboratory is designed to find any of the hundreds of

Type of Cancer	Per Year Risk (%)	Lifetime Risk (%)
Ductal or lobular	0.5–1.0	12–20
Ductal or lobular with associated LCIS/ALH	1.5–2.0	30
BRCA-1	5–10	50+

TABLE 15.2

Breast cancer incidence for high-risk women

different mutations in these genes that have been described. (Its name and number are listed in the "Resources" section of this book.) In addition, other laboratories offer testing for three specific mutations that are found in individuals of Ashkenazic ancestry (Jews of eastern Europe).

Clearly, the ability to identify women at increased risk for both ovarian and breast cancer will be helpful in our surveillance and prevention of these diseases. A government panel has recommended that women with mutations in BRCA-1 and BRCA-2 undergo surveillance for breast and ovarian cancer beginning before age thirty-five. This would include monthly breast self-examination, annual or semiannual clinician evaluation, and annual mammography. In addition, the drug tamoxifen (see chapter 11) may be considered to reduce the risk of breast cancer in women with mutations in these genes. A minority of women with hereditary risk choose surgical removal of the breast (prophylactic mastectomy), which has been shown to reduce the risk of breast cancer by 90 percent.

Women with mutations in BRCA-1 and BRCA-2 may also choose to undergo surveillance for ovarian cancer. Screening methods include ultrasound using an introvaginal probe and a blood test called CA 125, although neither of these methods has been shown to be very effective at finding ovarian cancer in its early stages. There are medications that may reduce the risk of ovarian cancer, however. For example, a recent study demonstrated that women with mutations who had taken birth control pills for approximately five years were far less likely to develop ovarian cancer. Finally, surgical removal of the ovaries may be considered, usually after age thirty-five or after childbearing is completed. Like prophylactic mastectomy, this procedure reduces but does not eliminate the risk of the disease.

CHECKPOINTS

1. If I assess my family history and determine that BRCA-1 is a possibility, what course of action is recommended? (You and your first-

degree relatives—siblings, mother, children—may want to undergo risk counseling and have a surveillance plan.)

2. What is my risk of a second breast cancer? Was there any lobular neoplasia in my biopsy?

3. If my family history is suggestive of hereditary breast cancer, would gene testing be helpful in decision making?

16

· · · · · ·

Fear of Recurrence

For those of you who are just starting the journey, you may want to put a note in your journal to revisit this chapter, since you most likely will be preoccupied with the current treatment of your breast cancer and can't even begin to think of a recurrence at this moment. However, if your cancer treatment is completed and you feel an unexplainable anxiety even though your trials are apparently over, read on.

These feelings are common and occur, in part, because the end has come to the frequent visits with your various doctors, which can serve to comfort—giving you the tangible evidence that someone is watching over you and your health. But, aside from that, you may be struggling with the fear of recurrence that many women experience at this time. Remember, during the treatment planning process, you want to develop a plan to optimize your chance of cure and to carry out that plan. When done, it is time for you to go on with your life. For some women, this means putting the whole process behind them, not allowing the experience even to enter their thoughts. But, for many women, life cannot ever be the same again. These women feel that they must do something to give the cancer meaning in their overall life experience—such as becoming an advocate for other women who may be suffering. Breast cancer enables major changes to take place in your life, whether they come in the form of helping a new friend or whatever other activity may create that meaning or sense of purpose for you. But, whatever you do, it is important to leave as much of your fear of cancer behind as possible.

Once a woman has breast cancer, there is an underlying fear of recurrence. A patient of mine once said, "Don't you realize you are never cured?" I said, "No, that's not true; women are most often cured, but none are ever absolutely sure." Unfortunately, some women do have recurrences, even after they have done everything they are supposed to do to prevent this.

But once you and your treatment team have done the best job possible, you must commit to continue on. Although this may be difficult initially, it becomes easier as time passes. I am often asked how a cure is defined. "Is it five years or ten years without recurrence?" The truth is that there is no magic length of time, although each of these anniversaries is very welcome to any breast cancer patient and her doctors. If a woman's cancer is destined to recur, over 75 percent will do so in the first five years following diagnosis and over 90 percent will recur at ten years.

There is tremendous controversy regarding how much and what kind of surveillance is necessary following the treatment of breast cancer. How closely should you be followed for recurrence and by whom? Since you are most likely being treated by several team members (surgeon, radiation oncologist, and medical oncologist), once your treatment is complete, you should discuss with your team who is the leader and who will order future tests for you.

At the least, you should be examined by a physician, usually the same examiner, every six months. If breast conservation with radiation, or lumpectomy alone, has been your local treatment, I recommend that you have a mammogram approximately six months after completion of your radiation or surgery. This serves as a new baseline that future test results can be measured against. You should then have a mammogram repeated on an annual basis. If you have had a mastectomy with or without reconstruction, the tissues just beneath the skin and axilla (armpit) are the areas of possible local recurrence, and a physical exam is all that is necessary for follow-up in your case. Although rare, it is important to discover *local* recurrence as soon as possible, and that is what these guidelines I am sharing are aimed at doing.

There is also controversy about how much testing is necessary to look for a systemic relapse. If you are on protocols testing new drug regimes, there may be set schedules for doing blood work, chest X rays, and bone scans. I don't recommend performing bone scans, CT scans, MRIs, et cetera, as routine follow-up if you are asymptomatic (without symptoms) because (1) these tests are expensive; (2) they expose you to radiation; and (3) studies show that finding a systemic recurrence a few months early, as these tests allow you to do, does not affect your further treatment or response.

Some oncologists order periodic blood tests that can reveal abnormalities with bone and liver function. There are also several markers in the blood that often rise with systemic recurrence, and which doctors can measure. Two marker blood tests that physicians widely use are the carcinoembryonic antigen (CEA) and the CA 27.29, also known as CA 15-3. Although the policy at our centers has been to order these blood tests every six months, I have a certain amount of ambivalence about this. My experience has been that a clear, incremental rise in the CEA or the CA 27.29 usually means impending systemic relapse with metastatic disease. Presently, my philosophy and approach for women with systemic relapse is palliation, which primarily deals with treating symptoms, prolonging life, and optimizing quality of life. It is difficult to treat a woman with systemic chemotherapy when she is asymptomatic except for an abnormal blood test and the quality of her life is excellent.

As part of everyday living and aging, we all experience a certain amount of achiness and fleeting intermittent body pains. Once you've been diagnosed with breast cancer, every new ache and pain can bring up the fear of recurrence. I suspect no woman ever completely gets over this fear, but time seems to make it more bearable. My general rule is for you to regard any new ache or pain for what it probably is: an ache or pain not related to recurrent breast cancer. Treatment is usually a mild anti-inflammatory and the tincture of time. If a pain persists and increases over a three- to four-week period, then it is probably important for you to see your doctor. However, even with this rule, it might be helpful for you to know that a majority of the more significant pains still turn out to be unrelated to the cancer.

It is very important to discuss follow-up with your physicians. Determine who is in charge and what is to be done in the years to come. Your return visits to your doctor, which once were a comfort, now can be traumatic because of their association with past heartache and pain. Knowing what to expect helps. Is it acceptable to be followed by your primary care physician only? I think so, as long as he or she is comfortable doing thorough examinations for local recurrence.

Once you have had breast cancer, you join a large group of women, well over 2 million strong, who are survivors. Your life will have changed in many ways forever. The way you choose to cope with being a survivor and meeting the fear of recurrence head-on will greatly influence the quality of the rest of your life.

CHECKPOINTS

1. Who is in charge of my surveillance after the end of treatment?
2. What is my checkup schedule? Does this change from year to year?
3. What tests should I expect to have at my checkup?

17

Hormone Replacement
after Breast Cancer

Hormone replacement therapy (HRT) is a major area of concern among women with a history of breast cancer. If you are in the crisis of a recent breast cancer diagnosis, the issue of HRT may seem relatively unimportant. However, as you get farther along and finish your treatment and proceed with your life, questions regarding HRT will certainly arise. I include this chapter here for you to review when you are ready.

Much has been written on the issue of HRT in general. Less is known specifically about HRT for breast cancer survivors because doctors have been concerned about prescribing anything for their patients that may increase the risk of recurrent disease. However, new research suggests this traditional tendency not to prescribe HRT for breast cancer survivors needs to be reevaluated. But, along with this, I must say blanket statements regarding HRT are not appropriate. Each individual woman must consider the risks and benefits of HRT based on her personal situation. Each woman experiences menopause differently, with varying degrees of symptoms. Some women ease into menopause with little problem and without increased risk of osteoporosis or heart disease. The menopause experience for others is traumatic and can introduce increased chances of illness into their lives.

The medical profession has endorsed allowing women to replace ovarian hormones with HRT once the ovaries begin to fail. Evidence and clinical experience indicate that the benefits clearly outweigh the risks and expense of such therapy. However, we do not have evidence of the risks to women surviving breast cancer. Our concerns are based on speculation and anecdotal experience alone.

For most women, the question is the relationship between HRT and an increased risk of breast cancer. Does hormone replacement contribute to breast cancer? At least twenty-four different studies and two meta-analyses (combining similar small studies to give greater statistical power) fail to show a causal relationship between the two. Researchers found no difference in breast cancer incidence for those women taking HRT and those women who did not in studies that controlled mammographic screening. Before starting HRT, physicians often require their patients to get a baseline screening mammogram, and because women receiving HRT are under a physician's surveillance, they are more likely to continue to get annual screenings. These women detect early cancer years before women not on HRT, who are less likely to get mammograms. If a researcher looks at breast cancer incidence over a short span of time, he/she may incorrectly conclude that HRT is responsible for an increased number of breast cancers when it is actually a case of early detection due to regular mammographic screening. Although there is no difference between women not taking HRT and those taking HRT for less than ten years, once the duration exceeds the ten-year mark, there is a slight increase in breast cancer incidence, but the numbers are small. There also appears to be anecdotal data that women with lobular neoplasia, either lobular cancer in situ (LCIS) or atypical lobular hyperplasia, may have an increased risk for recurrence with HRT. As we discussed previously, however, these women are at an increased risk regardless of hormone replacement usage.

Research has led us to conclude that low-dose HRT for less than ten years does not significantly contribute to the development of breast cancer in the general population. Does this apply to the population of women cured of breast cancer? Unfortunately, there are no studies to tell us this, and we do not know the answer. My own opinion is that for women with a high probability of cure, the benefits of HRT outweigh the risks.

How do you know you are cured, however? Unfortunately, there is no absolute way to know. We can give a statistical probability based on your cancer's characteristics. If you are destined to relapse, it will usually happen in the first five years after diagnosis. Unfortunately, late recurrences do rarely occur. I advise my patients that once treatment is complete, they should consider themselves cured and move on. Granted, they are never the same and there is that "gray cloud on the horizon," but the cloud becomes smaller as time passes.

Women often ask me, "But what if I'm not cured? Can HRT cause increased harm?" I don't know the answer to this, either. Theoretically, HRT could stimulate cells that have escaped systemically and stimulate them to grow and appear more rapidly. On the other hand, if this were to happen, tamoxifen or one of the newer hormonal therapies should then make the cancer regress.

We have only roundabout evidence regarding HRT in breast cancer survivors. For example, we know that younger women who have had breast cancer and then go on to become pregnant, with the associated high levels of estrogen and progesterone, do not have a worse prognosis or earlier relapse of breast cancer than women who do not experience a pregnancy. If estrogen can theoretically stimulate breast cancer growth, why do we see breast cancer appear in older postmenopausal women who are not on HRT? This is a fairly frequent occurrence, and most of these cancers are hormone receptor positive, yet they are growing in an estrogen-poor environment. This seems to counter what we know about the environment that is conducive to breast cancer, but this is just another reminder of how much we do not understand about this disease.

In most cases, if a young premenopausal woman with hormone receptor positive breast cancer is given tamoxifen, the cancer will get smaller and regress. At the same time, the tamoxifen will cause the woman's blood estrogen levels to increase. The cancer must have a higher affinity to tamoxifen than to estrogen in order for the drug to be effective. In spite of high estrogen levels, the tamoxifen works to kill the cancer. Is it then possible to give both HRT and tamoxifen together and get the benefits of each?

Doctors have prescribed this dual treatment in the United Kingdom without reported ill effects, but American oncologists have been very hesitant to do this routinely without longer experience to assess risk of recurrence. What is needed is a clinical trial comparing HRT versus HRT plus tamoxifen versus tamoxifen alone versus no hormonal treatment. Such a trial, unfortunately, would take large numbers of women, and some of these women would have to participate on a no-treatment "arm," or protocol. That has yet to be done. Researchers are also diligently working on new SERMs that are less stimulatory to the uterus and may potentially relieve menopausal symptoms while maintaining the ability to kill cancer cells. If such a new drug is found, there will be no need to administer both HRT and tamoxifen.

Let's put the theoretical data to work for us and look at what to do with the information at hand. Are the benefits of HRT for the breast cancer survivor adequate to outweigh the theoretical risks? This is obviously not an easy question, and each individual woman's situation is quite different in regard to it. Some factors for you to consider are your

- risk of recurrence
- type of breast cancer (presence of lobular neoplasia and hormone receptors)
- risk of heart disease
- cholesterol and lipoprotein levels
- risk of osteoporosis
- bone mineral density
- risk of uterine cancer
- quality-of-life issues (libido, vaginal atrophy, hot flashes, depression, memory loss)
- risk of Alzheimer's disease (Some recent intriguing reports indicate

that HRT may prevent Alzheimer's. Although very preliminary, this new information perhaps should also be factored into the equation.)

I suggest you meet with your oncologist and discuss the risks and benefits of HRT in your individual situation based on the above factors. If you and your doctor make the joint decision that you take HRT, the question then becomes whether there is one preparation that is better than another.

Here again, we face the problem of lack of evidence and controlled studies as we make these decisions. The literature indicates that different estrogen preparations stimulate the ductal glandular tissue to varying degrees. Estradiol is much more stimulatory than estriol. The most commonly used preparation, Premarin, is primarily estriol and appears to benefit bones and lower cholesterol. The unanswered question is, What is the benefit of adding tamoxifen to HRT? For women who have a uterus, the addition of low-dose progesterone appears to protect against uterine cancer.

A new SERM, raloxifene hydrochloride (Evista), has been approved in the United States for the treatment of osteoporosis. Raloxifene does not appear to stimulate the uterine lining, nor does it appear to stimulate breast glandular tissue to activate. Presently, it is being tested against tamoxifen as a breast cancer prevention therapy. Breast cancer survivors who have completed therapy and are concerned about osteoporosis and heart disease might consider raloxifene hydrochloride as an alternative to HRT. Unfortunately raloxifene hydrochloride does not usually alleviate menopausal symptoms such as hot flashes and vaginal dryness. This is something you should discuss with your oncologist. As I mentioned earlier, the pharmaceutical industry is striving to produce the "perfect" SERM. Until then, one must weigh the risks and benefits of what is available.

CHECKPOINTS

1. What are the specific risk factors, if any, for taking hormone replacement in my case?
2. What is my family history of breast, ovarian, and uterine cancer?
3. How long should I wait after my initial treatment before I begin to consider HRT?
4. Are natural hormones available?

18

How to Work
the Medical System

In this chapter I hope to provide you with some helpful information about how to get your cancer treatment accomplished effectively within the medical system. There is nothing more distressing than being diagnosed with cancer and then having to deal with an environment that is intimidating and foreign at the same time. Many find this combination simply overwhelming. Your task is further complicated by the fact that you will need to see a number of physicians, requiring you to deal with several different offices and treatment facilities at the same time.

Although sometimes it may not seem this way, the medical system in the United States is composed mostly of compassionate people who have chosen this field of work because they want to help others. Taking care of cancer patients has wonderful rewards, but it also presents a great deal of stress and frustration to its practitioners. The practice of medicine is changing dramatically, particularly in regard to the increasing amount of paperwork and bureaucratic hassle doctors and nurses face with the changing role of insurance and HMOs.

So, my first suggestion to you is *be pleasant and patient, but persistent.* Second, it is important to remember that on the other end of the phone or across the desk is a real person. *Write down each person's name* you speak to, and make an attempt to remember it if you are going to be dealing with him or her in the future. Personal connections are beneficial and help to alleviate distress as you work your way through your diagnosis and treatment plan.

Every office and treatment facility has key individuals you will need to get to know. There is usually a clinical person who has the physician's ear and a key business person who can assist you with insurance problems and authorization procedures. Many patients don't understand how to employ the help of these key individuals and incidentally bypass them. Physicians do not want to deal with the business aspects of your treatment, such as speaking to or coordinating with insurance companies and managed care organizations, unless they absolutely have to. Most of these issues can be solved by their specialized personnel whose job it is to do so.

For your questions or problems that arise between scheduled office visits, you should have a nurse specialist or paramedical person to talk to. It is important to go to this person first. You may want to talk to your doctor directly, but it is wiser not to bypass this assigned person. For if you bypass this individual, he or she will have no opportunity to assist you and serve as your advocate—now or in the future. In the worst-case scenario, you could need emergency help and he or she might not be aware of important medical information concerning your case. In addition, if you go directly to your physician with nonmedical issues or medical questions the staff could handle, you may find him or her resistant or frustrated and not as eager to talk to you in the future. This you should try to avoid.

You want to utilize each person at each medical office you deal with in the most appropriate manner possible and not alienate anyone by not doing so. But how are you to know when and to whom you should bring your concerns? My suggestion is to always direct your question at the staff, even if it is urgent or an emergency, and let them help you first. They can get to the physician faster than you can, if need be, and will know when to do just that. To address key specific issues with your doctor personally, go in to his or her office with a list of your concerns and questions simply and directly stated. In the next chapter we will discuss keeping a personal log, which should aid you in this process.

If you seem to be having a communication problem with one of your treating physicians, speak directly to him or her first to attempt to resolve the situation. If you cannot get results this way, you may need to go for help to your primary care physician or the physician you have chosen to be your coordinator. Remember: *Be pleasant and patient, but persistent.* If you are dealing with an HMO and are having trouble with the system, you do have options. This is when it pays to be a *squeaky wheel.* You need to document your problem and then take it up the ladder, as high as you need to go to get it addressed. In these organizations, as in most hospitals, there is an administrative ladder and a medical ladder. At the top is the CEO of the organization and a medical director. Both directors have phones, mail boxes, fax numbers, and E-mail. Although you may not have to take an issue you are wrestling with that far, it may be helpful to know someone is, eventually, accountable and that you can reach that person.

With all the recent changes in health care and the complexity of the treatment of breast cancer, there is great potential for problems of coordination and communication. Remember that whether you pay cash for your care or belong to an HMO, you are a purchaser of health care and have choices and rights. Each HMO is required to have, in writing, its policy and procedure for grievances and disputes. You have a right to this information and should follow it, taking your complaint step-by-step as far as it needs to go to be resolved.

In the face of a new diagnosis of breast cancer and the need to educate yourself and explore options, it can be difficult to navigate the medical bureaucracy alone. After all, you have only so much time and physical and emotional energy. It is helpful to have assistance with this process. A spouse, a sibling, a parent, a good friend, or a significant other can act as your primary advocate, if you like. I do not want you to become bogged down, tired, and discouraged, relinquishing control over your all-important treatment plan. If you feel this happening to you, ask for help! Some women have difficulty asking for help, and if you are reading this as a husband, sibling, or friend, your active participation can make a critical difference to the person you care about.

CHECKPOINTS

1. Remember: Be pleasant and patient, but persistent.
2. Always write down the name of the person you are dealing with and attempt to use and remember it.
3. Who is my advocate at my doctor's office, and how do I contact this person?
4. Who is my primary health care advocate, and what do I expect of him or her?

19

Logs and Calendars

Because the treatment of breast cancer is complex and can involve many doctors and treatment facilities, you run the risk of getting care that is fragmented and duplicated. Because of this fragmentation, innocent mistakes can occur that could affect your treatment or be frustrating for you. This is the outcome if your records are different at each facility and letters, test results, and other important information do not get to each doctor or treatment facility in a timely fashion. You want to do all you can to avoid such occurrences.

Some of my patients have addressed this problem by taking control of their own medical information. They have created a personal copy of all records from every doctor and treatment facility, which they keep in their own possession at all times. This can lead to better care and give you a greater sense of control over your treatment. I highly recommend it. If you make a point of collecting this information from the very beginning of your diagnosis and treatment, you will find it takes little extra effort to maintain your file. The Breast Center keeps an updated history report on every patient (see Figure 19.1); this is an example of the kind of report that would be beneficial for you to collect. Alert every office staff member that you want copies of any letters written or reports received in their office from the onset and follow up with

Patient:_____DOB:_____

Diagnosis Date:_____Type:_____T_____N_____M_____

Histology: BR_____ER_____PR_____Her2Neu_____

DNA:_____S-phase:_____

Surgeon(s), Surgery(ies) & Date(s):_____

_____

Chemotherapy Protocol(s) & Dates(s):_____

_____

Radiation Protocol(s) & Date(s):_____

_____

Hormone Therapy(ies) & Date(s):_____

_____

Miscellaneous:_____

_____

Primary Care Physician:_____Phone:_____

FAX:_____Contact Person:_____

Authorization needed: Office visits: yes/no   Chemotherapy: yes/no

FIGURE 19.1
The Breast Center's patient history report form

them regularly, checking in for new information with a friendly reminder. Do not let anyone give you a hard time with this. *You have a legal right to your records.*

The advantages of possessing your own records are obvious. At any given encounter with a doctor, you have all of your information in hand. It also sends a message to your team that you want to be involved.

Organizing Your Medical Information

✺ I suggest you adopt an organized approach to collecting your medical information from the time you are diagnosed with breast cancer. Purchase a three-ring binder with dividers, and create the following categories:

1. *Insurance/doctor directory.* This section includes such personal information as your insurance policy number and the address and phone number of your insurance company, your date of birth and social security number as well as those of your spouse, work phone numbers, people to call in an emergency and their numbers, baby-sitters, and anyone whose phone numbers and addresses you may need in a pinch. The section should also list the names, office addresses, phone numbers, and fax numbers of all your physicians, present and past. You can collect business cards and paste or tape them to the pages. These can then be copied and given to the various offices for your permanent patient file.

2. *Reports.* Collect operative reports from all surgeries and the pathology reports on tissue as outlined in chapter 4. If an assay is performed as to which chemotherapy drugs your cancer is sensitive to, put that information in this section as well.

3. *Consultations and letters.* Include letters from one physician to another. Also place in this section any second opinion conference summaries you obtain.

4. *Lab work and test results.* Include reports of blood work, mammograms, X rays, and bone scans.

5. *Calendar.* This can be either an independent section or placed in the first section with your basic information. A one-year calendar on a single page works well, for it allows you to see, at a glance, the overall progress of your treatment. It also permits you to observe the larger picture of how your surgery is sequenced with radiation and/or chemotherapy. Another advantage of a calendar is that it allows you to make plans for vacations, business trips, and other obligations between treatments. See Figure 19.2 for a sample 1998 calendar.

6. *An ongoing log.* Maintain a diary of events related to your treatment. You can include medications, visits to doctors, and treatments. You can also record your symptoms here and make notes about events. This information will help when you visit your doctors and they ask you specific questions about your treatment history and your response to it.

7. *Insurance and financial data.* In this section you can include bills, statements, explanation of benefits (EOB), payment records, et cetera.

8. *Goals and changes.* This is an optional category. A diagnosis of cancer sometimes prompts one to take a good look at one's life. The first six months of a breast cancer diagnosis usually involve juggling treatment with everyday tasks. All too often, once treatment is done, it's back to business as usual for you. Your intentions to change and new goals often go on hold. But many women do make important and meaningful changes in their lives after gaining profound insights as a result of their battle with breast cancer.

   I suggest that you set down five to ten goals or changes for your life and assume you will have at least five healthy years to make them. Why only five years? Because that time line does not give you time to procrastinate, and you will make changes that translate quickly into results. Ending an addictive relationship,

1998

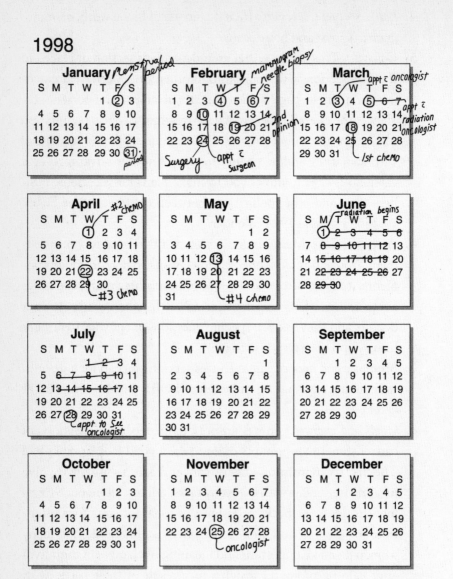

FIGURE **19.2**

A sample calendar for organizing medical information

planting an exotic flower garden, taking the vacation you have been postponing, writing that book, or embracing new and exciting risks are some examples of the types of changes I have seen my patients make as a result of the goals they've set. The transformations that can occur as a result of triumphing over something as challenging as breast cancer are wondrous to observe. Sometimes, as a breast cancer specialist, they are what keeps me inspired to continue my work.

Tape-Recording Medical Sessions

At our breast center, we automatically tape-record every consultation and second opinion session, and give the tape to each patient. We understand that an extensive amount of information is exchanged that you may not remember because of your fear, stress, and anxiety. Some physicians are uncomfortable allowing tape-recording of visits, and I recommend that you kindly but persistently ask for the right to tape at important sessions. If your significant other cannot attend, then you have an accurate accounting to share later. Many misunderstandings can be cleared up by reviewing the taped material again. Will the tape recorder change the content or conduct of the meeting between you and your physician? In my own experience, *no*. It does not make a difference if a recorder is present or not.

Keeping a Journal

The process of writing down your experiences and feelings can be very beneficial and healing. A patient of mine, Cathy Moore, and her good friend Robin Bernstein are the authors of a book called *Journal for Healing* (Main Street Books, Doubleday), which deals with journal writing during an illness. They make some wonderful points regarding the short- and long-term benefits of recording your experiences. It is a way to express yourself without fear of consequences.

CHECKPOINTS

1. Ask my physician's office staff to give me copies of all correspondence, blood work, and reports. Ask them to put a notation in my medical record file for future reference.
2. Purchase a binder and organize dividers.

Conclusion
More about This Manual

The diagnosis of breast cancer forces a life crisis. For each woman, the crisis is as different as her life is. For most, there are the questions of *why* and *how*. Questions to which there are no real answers. Ahead, you have an unchosen, unavoidable path full of decisions and some unpleasant tasks. Many describe the most troublesome aspect of their ordeal with breast cancer as the anxiety of the unknown. This manual should set you off on your journey with more of the knowledge and direction you desire.

There are tremendous monetary and human resources being devoted to discovering the cause(s) and cure of breast cancer. This process will continue as you start and progress on your journey. You may need to modify your path based on information revealed by new discoveries. Presently, however, you must make decisions based on what is the best information at hand. Your choices may include taking some risks and experiencing some unpleasant effects of treatment for the trade-off of an increased chance of cure.

How do you keep as informed as possible about new developments? Remember: This is a disease that affects one in every nine women. New developments are newsworthy. You will probably find that you are now suddenly aware of developments in cancer research and particularly breast cancer in the news media. Your doctors will be receiving information on a professional level through their journals and meetings that they will share with you as well. Try to let everyone in your treatment team know you are interested in information, and keep your eyes open for it—in whatever periodicals you read, on TV, and through the Internet.

You should know that most women today are cured of breast cancer. They undergo treatment, become survivors, and go on with their lives. But having cancer is certainly a wake-up call to many and may be for you. Life now has added uncertainty. There exists an eminent, nagging cloud on the horizon. As I have discussed in this manual, some women capitalize on the crisis. They use it to transform their lives. Some tear the house down, so to speak, while others simply remodel. Breast cancer makes you painfully aware of your vulnerability and your mortality, but there is value added—a richness, a deeper sensitivity, an appreciation of life and beauty, and, for some, a motivation to transform. Many women find they are stronger than they ever imagined.

Some of the information in this manual will rapidly become outdated and replaced by newer data, but the philosophy I have espoused and shared with you will always hold true. This philosophy is that you must become critically involved in your care and the decision-making process regarding your treatment. Since we, the medical profession, are asking you to enter into the decision-making process, you must be educated about your individual situation and the risks and benefits of treatment options. The treatment directed at your cancer involves you as a whole person—in the physical, psychological, and spiritual sense.

The crisis of breast cancer is unfortunately all too common. It is an unchosen journey with some uncertainties and potential opportunities. I hope this manual will get you started and help you navigate the way in the most positive and educated manner possible. *Good luck!*

Resources

These resources can help you get started gathering information and facts about cancer.

Organizations

American Cancer Society
1 (800) 227-2345 has a variety of breast cancer services including *Special Touch*, a breast health program teaching breast self-examination (BSE), and *Reach to Recovery*, a support program for women initially diagnosed with breast cancer. *Look Good . . . Feel Better* is a program designed to help women with their appearance.

American College of Radiology
1 (800) 227-5463 can provide a list of accredited facilities for mammography in your area.

American Society of Plastic and Reconstructive Surgeons (ASPRS)
1 (800) 635-0635 provides a list of board-certified physicians in your area.

The Breast Cancer Fund
1 (800) 487-0492 is a national nonprofit organization that supports cutting-edge research, education, patient support, and advocacy projects through highly visible efforts such as *Expedition Inspiration*, a mountain climb by a team of breast cancer survivors.

Cancer Care, Inc.
1 (800) 813-4673, 1 (800) 813-HOPE, provides free professional counseling and referral services.

ICI Pharmaceutical Nolvadex Patient Assistance Program
1 (800) 456-5678 will help financially eligible women receive tamoxifen.

International Cancer Alliance (ICA)
1 (800) 422-7361, 1 (800) I CARE 61, provides a *Cancer Therapy Review* that includes information about cancer and clinical trials.

Myriad Genetics, Inc.
1 (800) 469-7423 provides testing for BRCA-1 and BRCA-2 (Web site: http://www.myriad.com).

National Alliance of Breast Cancer Organizations (NABCO)
1 (800) 719-9154 is a national organization providing information on breast cancer targeting increased research funding.

National Black Leadership Initiative on Cancer (NBLIC)
1 (800) 262-5420 provides community outreach for African-American women, including screening services and access to health care systems.

National Breast Cancer Coalition (NBCC)
1 (202) 296-7477 is a nationwide lobbyist organization for increased funding for breast cancer research.

National Cancer Institute (NCI) Information Service
1 (800) 4-CANCER is a national Cancer Information Service (CIS). CIS serves as a community resource and provides information about cancer, includ-

ing NCI's treatment database. The NCI also organizes the Physician Data Query (PDQ), which gives information on clinical trials.

National Lymphedema Network
1 (800) 541-3259 provides information about the prevention and treatment of lymphedema.

Oncotech
1 (800) 662-6832 provides testing of cancer cells for drug resistance and sensitivity.

Rational Therapeutics Cancer Laboratories
1 (562) 989-6455 is a cancer evaluation center that provides testing of cancer cells for drug resistance and sensitivity (E-Mail: RationalT@aol.com, Website: http//www.rational-t.com).

Single Point of Contact (SPOC)
1 (888) 249-4918 provides help from Genentech Oncology in getting Herceptin authorized by your insurance company or will provide your oncologist with drug for free if you qualify for their patient assistance program.

Susan G. Komen Breast Cancer Foundation
1 (800) 462-9273, 1 (800) I'M AWARE, supports research, education, and treatment of breast cancer. Free screenings, breast exam, and BSE instruction are available for seniors and women with limited resources. The foundation is also an annual sponsor of *Race for the Cure*, a 5/10K run/walk to raise money for breast cancer.

Weisenthal Cancer Group
1 (714) 894-0011 provides diagnostic analysis of cancer tissue and information on recommended chemotherapeutic agents.

Y-ME National Organization for Breast Cancer
1 (800) 221-2141 is a nonprofit organization providing information, telephone counseling, educational programs, and support groups for breast cancer survivors and their families.

Internet

The Internet is changing daily, and information and access numbers can become obsolete before you know it. You may want to consult the Internet directories available at your local library. One problem with the Internet is finding not too little information but too much. Another problem is that the information you get from the Internet can be inaccurate. It is necessary to distinguish between personal Web sites and official Web sites of bona fide, reputable organizations. This is not always easy to do. The following suggestions should help you get started and, I hope, lead you quickly to the right information for you.

The fastest way to get a clickable listing of URLs on breast cancer is through a search program such as Alta Vista: http://altavista.digital.com/. Probably the single best link is http://wwwicic.nci.nih.gov/. This gives you the National Cancer Institute and the International Cancer Information Center at the National Institutes of Health. Whether you're a patient, health professional, or researcher, you'll find your links here. You'll get up-to-date information and phone numbers too. The New York Breast Cancer Information Clearing House at http://nysernet.ort/bcic offers you another perspective. Type in http://www.nlm.nih.gov/ and you will find the U.S. National Library of Medicine. One of the nice things you can do here is a free search of MEDLINE data, for those interested in abstracts of scientific articles on breast cancer and other topics.

Other useful Web sites for information on cancer are:

- BreastCancer.Net (www.breastcancer.net). You can get a daily E-mail highlighting all the day's new breast cancer articles on the WWW.
- CancerOnline (http://www.stonecottage.com/canceronline/)
- OncoLink® (http://www.oncolink.upenn.edu/)
- Dr. C. Everett Koop, former U.S. surgeon general, has a very informative Web site (http://drkoop.com).

Finally, there is our center's very own Web page, http://www.breastlinkcare.com. We invite you to come and visit us.

We also have a nonprofit organization, Breast Cancer Care & Research Fund, which is developing its own Web site at (http://www.breastcancercare.org). Our goal is to empower you with information that is up-to-date, accurate and, most importantly, relevant. The Web site is uniquely devoted only to breast cancer and does not receive any funding from drug companies, hospitals, physician groups, or any other source that could possibly compromise our mission of providing honest, unbiased information. We hope you check our site frequently for the most current, accurate, and unbiased source of news on breast cancer on the Internet.

Glossary

acute: Sharp, intense, and of short duration.

adjuvant: Auxiliary, an aid to remove or prevent disease.

allergen: Any substance that causes manifestations of allergies (abnormal and individual hypersensitivity to substances that are ordinarily harmless).

alopecia: Absence or loss of hair.

amino acids: The building blocks of proteins and the end products of protein digestion.

ancillary: Additional, auxiliary.

aneuploid: Cells with an atypical amount of DNA.

angiogenesis: Development of blood vessels.

apoptosis: Disintegration of cells into membrane-bound particles that are destroyed by other cells.

areola: A circular pigmented area around the breast nipple.

assay: Analysis of a substance.

asymptomatic: Without symptoms.

atypia: Change in a cell that suggests a tendency toward malignant transformation.

atypical: Not conforming to a regular type.

atypical lobular hyperplasia: Abnormally shaped cells proliferating excessively in the normal tissue arrangement of a breast lobule.

autosomal dominant gene: Non-sex-based gene that requires only one copy in order to be expressed.

autosomal recessive gene: Non-sex-based gene that requires two copies in order to be expressed.

autosome: Any chromosome other than a sex chromosome.

axillary lymph nodes: Lymph nodes in the armpit.

basement membrane: The separating membrane of the cell that provides a boundary from adjacent tissue.

biopsy: Excision of a small piece of living tissue for microscopic examination; usually performed to establish a diagnosis.

blue node: The first lymph node that stains blue after injection of blue dye into a tumor and its surrounding tissue.

BMT: bone marrow transplant.

bone marrow rescue: The preservation of the soft organic material that fills the bone cavity; used after administration of high-dose chemotherapy.

carcinoembryonic antigens (CEA): A class of antigens normally present in the fetus; originally isolated from colon tumors. If the previously elevated CEA levels return to normal after surgery, it is thought to indicate complete tumor removal.

catechol estrogen: A form of estrogen that is biologically unavailable.

chronic: Of long duration.

clear margin: Surrounding area of tissue that is clear of cancer cells after surgery.

clinical stage: Denoting diagnosis and treatment on the basis of observation, pathology, and symptoms of patients.

colloid cancer: A rare ductal cancer also known as mucinous cancer.

combination chemotherapy: Combining drugs together in a single treatment.

cribiform: A pattern of cancer cell growth inside the breast duct that resembles mesh.

cytosarcoma phylloides: A tumor of the breast that is of nonepithelial origin.

cytotoxic agents: Chemicals that destroy cells or prevent their multiplication.

daughter cell: The product of cell division.

dermis: The layer of tissue under the outer skin.

diffuse: Spreading, scattered.

diploid: Having two sets of chromosomes.

disease: The lack of ease; a pathological condition of the body.

dose intensification: Intensifying the administration of chemotherapy by increasing the dose or shortening the time interval between treatments.

ductal cancer in situ (DCIS): A cancer encapsulated within the breast ducts.

ductal cell: A cell from the duct of the breast.

electron beam boost: Use of radioactive particles to target a specific area of the body with additional radiation treatments.

empirical: Based on practical experience but not proven scientifically.

endogenous estrogen: Estrogen that is produced within the body.

enzyme: An organic catalyst produced by living cells but capable of acting independently. Enzymes produce chemical changes without being changed themselves.

epithelium: Cells that form a barrier to underlying tissue such as skin, ducts, and glands.

estrogen: The female sex hormone produced by the ovary. Estrogens are responsible for the development of secondary sexual characteristics and for cyclic changes in the vaginal epithelium and endothelium of the uterus.

expander: A polyurethane flexible implant that is placed under the tissue and is enlarged manually by inserting a fluid, usually saline.

extracellular: Outside a cell or cells.

fluoropyrimidine: A class of compounds that act as false building blocks for DNA.

frank menopause: Obvious menopause.

free-radical damage: Damage to tissue by molecules containing an odd number of electrons.

frozen section: The thin cut of a frozen specimen for rapid examination of tissue by a pathologist.

gamma probe: A handheld instrument to detect areas of radioactive material.

genistein: A phytoestrogen produced by soy products.

haploid: Possessing half the diploid, or normal, number of chromosomes found in somatic cells.

HDC: High-dose chemotherapy.

Her-2/neu oncogene: An oncogene that is abnormally stimulated to produce an excess of protein, affecting cell division in the breast.

heterogeneous disease: A disease that does not manifest itself in the same way in every patient; having varying or dissimilar characteristics.

high-grade cancer: A cancer with a Bloom Richardson Grading Scale of 8 to 9, commonly with a high vascular component.

histamines: Substances that are released from target cells and that cause membrane secretions plus blood vessel dilatation. Chemotherapy stimulates massive histamine release from the upper gut, causing the nausea associated with treatment.

histologic grade: The microscopic measure and evaluation of the structure of a cancer.

holistic approach: Treatment that involves the entire body, including the mind and spirit.

homogeneous: Uniform in nature; a similar cause.

hormone: A substance that originates in a gland and that is conveyed through the blood to another part of the body, stimulating it by chemical action to increase functional activity or increase secretion of other hormones.

hyperplasia: An increase in the number of cells in the lining of a gland.

hypoglycemia: Deficiency of sugar in the blood.

hypothesis: An educated guess; a preliminary assumption based on enough observation to place it beyond mere speculation but requiring further experiments for verification.

in situ: In the normal place without disturbing the surrounding tissue, localized.

infiltrating lobular carcinoma: Cancerous cells in the breast lobule that have spread through the basement membrane into the surrounding breast tissue.

invasive cancer: Cancer cells that penetrate the basement membrane, resulting in spread to healthy tissue.

isoflavone: A chemical found in soy products.

liposarcoma: A cancer of the fat cell.

lobular carcinoma in situ (LCIS): A change in the breast lobule that increases risk of breast cancer. It is a marker for breast cancer.

lobular cell: A cell in the lobule of the breast; used for making milk.

lobular neoplasia: An abnormal accumulation of cells in the terminal lobule. When present, increases the risk of future breast cancer. Once called LCIS.

local control: The control of cancer in the breast.

local recurrence: The return of cancerous cells to the breast.

lumen: The space within a tube, vein, or artery.

lumpectomy: Surgical removal of a tumor from the breast to clear margins not including the lymph nodes; also known as a wide local excision.

lymphedema: Edema or swelling caused by obstruction of lymph channels.

lymph node: A rounded body consisting of an accumulation of lymphatic tissue found at intervals in the course of lymphatic vessels. Lymph nodes vary in size from a pinhead to an olive and can occur singularly or in groups. They produce lymphocytes and monocytes, and serve to filter matter from entering the bloodstream.

lymphocytes: Cells that travel in the bloodstream to and from the lymph nodes, providing the body with immune capability.

lymphoma: Tumor of the lymph tissue.

macroscopic: Visible to the naked eye; gross observation.

main tumor: A spontaneous new growth of tissue made up of abnormally dividing cells that form a mass.

markers: Blood tests that register tumor antigens.

mastitis: Inflammation or infection of the breast.

meiosis: The process during cell division when the diploid chromosome number becomes reduced to the haploid.

metastatic disease: Movement of cancer cells from one part of the body to another.

microinvasion: Invasion of cancer cells through the breast duct into adjacent tissue at a microscopic level.

microscopic focus: The starting point of a disease process.

mitochondria: The source of energy for a cell; involved with protein synthesis and lipid metabolism.

mitosis: The reproduction of cells; the process of cell division.

mitotic rate: Rate or speed of cell division.

mutation: Any basic alteration in form, quality, or some other characteristic. A change in genetic material of a chromosome that produces a new individual unlike its parents.

necrosis: Death of areas of tissue surrounded by healthy parts.

neoadjuvant chemotherapy: The use of chemotherapy prior to curative resection of malignancy.

neovascularization: The ability of a cancer to form new blood vessels.

neuropathy: Disease or damage of the nerves, causing lack of sensitivity or numbness.

neurotransmitters: Chemicals in the brain that relay messages from one neuron to another.

nuclear pleomorphism: More than one form of nuclei in various cells.

oncogene: A gene that has the ability to induce a cell to become malignant. In addition to genes that induce tumor formation, there are antioncogenes that suppress tumors.

oxidative burst: The rapid combination of a substance with oxygen.

palliation: The process of relieving without curing; alleviating discomfort and symptoms.

palpable: Capable of being touched or felt.

papillary cancer: A type of ductal cancer in the breast.

pathology report: An evaluation performed by a physician who specializes in the diagnosis of structural and functional changes in tissue that result from disease processes.

pedicle: A stem of tissue containing blood vessels allowing for the movement of that tissue to another area of the body.

perimenopausal: Around menopause.

phytoalexins: Substances produced by plants. These counteract plant infections.

phytochemicals: Chemicals found in plants.

phytoestrogens: An estrogenlike substance produced by plants.

pilot studies: Research investigations that explore a particular drug, technique, or idea.

placebo: Inactive substance given to patients as medicine; also used in control studies of drugs.

pleomorphic lobular cancer: A more aggressive form of lobular cancer.

ploidy: The number of chromosome sets in a cell, that is, haploidy, diploidy, triploidy (one, two, and three sets of chromosomes, respectively).

polyunsaturated fats: Fats made up of long-chain carbon compounds with many carbon atoms joined by double or triple bonds.

premalignant: Before metastasis; cancerous growth (as in LCIS).

pre-pectoral fascia: A tissue covering the pectoralis muscle that separates the breast tissue from the underlying muscle and acts as a natural barrier.

progesterone: A steroid hormone from the corpus leuteum and placenta. It is responsible for changes in the endometrium in the second half of the menstrual cycle, development of the maternal placenta, and development of the mammary glands.

prognostic factors: Factors influencing the prediction of the outcome of a disease.

prophylactic: Contributing to the prevention of infection or disease.

prosthesis: Artificial substitute for a missing part of the body.

quadrant: One quarter; the breast is divided into four quadrants: upper outer, upper inner, lower outer, and lower inner.

randomized clinical trial: An investigation of the effects of a drug administered to human subjects. The goal is to define the clinical efficiency and pharmacological effects (toxicity, side effects, interactions) of the substance. This is done by a random method of assigning subjects to experimental treatment or nontreatment groups.

receptors: A cell component that combines with a drug, hormone, or chemical mediator to alter the function of the cell.

reconstruction: The action of constructing again. In breast reconstruction, the surgically altered breast is returned to its approximate original state.

remission: The period when cancer appears to be inactive.

satellite nodules: Small structures attached to the larger tumor.

scatter damage: Damage caused to tissue by the diffusion of X rays when they strike an object.

sensitivity: The ability to react to stimuli. The value of a diagnostic test; the procedure of clinical observation.

sentinel node: The first lymph node draining a malignant tumor.

sequential chemotherapy: Using drugs in a singular manner, in a set sequence.

SERM: Selective estrogen receptor modulators.

simulation: Radiation planning session designed to map out the radiation field.

skin sparing mastectomy: A mastectomy that spares a majority of the skin overlying the removed breast tissue. Can be filled with tissue from a transfer or a silicone or saline implant.

S phase: A period of chromosome replication during mitosis.

sporadic: Occurring occasionally or at scattered intervals.

staging system: The assessment of a cancer by size and quality.

state of the art: The best treatment available.

stem cell: An immature blood cell that has the ability to generate new bone marrow.

synergistic: The combining of drugs that may enhance the positive effect over what would be achieved by giving the drugs alone, in sequence.

systemic control: The control of cancer throughout the body.

systemic spread: The spread of cancer cells to the other organs via the bloodstream.

tissue transfer: Breast reconstruction by removing tissue from other parts of the body and replacing it in the breast.

toxicity: The extent or degree of being poisonous.

transient: Of brief duration.

transient menopause: Rapid onset of menopause caused by chemotherapy.

transverse rectus abdominis mycutaneous (TRAM) flap: Breast reconstruction surgery that uses tissue from the abdomen to rebuild the breast.

treatment arm: A selected treatment group.

tubular cancer: A slow growing, rare type of ductal cancer.

vascular system: The heart, blood vessels, lymphatics, and their parts considered collectively.

vasculitis: Inflammation of a blood or lymph vessel.

wide local excision (WLE): See lumpectomy.

Index